THE HEALTHCARE EXECUTIVE'S GUIDE TO PHYSICIAN-HOSPITAL ALIGNMENT

COKER GROUP

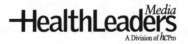

┼HCPro

Coker Group, Author
Karen Kondilis, Editor
Bob Wertz, Editorial Director
Matt Cann, Group Publisher
Jim DeWolf, Editorial Director

Doug Ponte, Cover Designer
Mike Mirabello, Graphic Artist
Matt Sharpe, Production Manager
Shane Katz, Art Director
Jean St. Pierre, Vice President of Operations

Advice given is general. Readers should consult professional counsel for specific legal, ethical, or clinical questions. Arrangements can be made for quantity discounts. For more information, contact:

HCPro, Inc.
75 Sylvan Street, Suite A-101
Danvers, MA 01923
Telephone: 800-650-6787 or 781-639-1872
Fax: 800-639-8511
Email: *customerservice@hcpro.com*

HCPro, Inc., is the parent company of HealthLeaders Media.

Visit HealthLeaders Media online at *www.healthleadersmedia.com*

03/2013
22011

Contents

Contents

Contents

About the Author

Max Reiboldt, CPA

Max Reiboldt provides sound financial and strategic solutions to hospitals, medical practices, health systems, and other healthcare entities through keen analysis and problem solving. Working with organizations of all sizes, Reiboldt engages in consulting projects with organizations nationwide. His expertise encompasses employee and physician employment and compensation, physician/hospital affiliation initiatives, business and strategic planning, mergers and acquisitions, practice operational assessments, ancillary services development, PHO/IPA/MSO development, practice appraisals, and negotiations for acquisitions and sales. He also performs financial analyses for healthcare entities as well as buy/sell agreements and planning arrangements for medical practices.

Reiboldt is president and CEO of Coker Group and has led the firm's growth since the late 1990s to its position today as one of the leading healthcare consulting firms in the United States and abroad. He is a prolific author and accomplished public speaker on healthcare management topics.

Reiboldt has authored or contributed to many of Coker Group's 60-plus books. Recent titles include *Financial Management of the Medical Practice*, Third Edition (©2011, AMA Press), *Reimbursement Management: Improving the*

Success and Profitability of Your Practice (©2011, AMA Press), *RVUs at Work: Relative Value Units in the Medical Practice* (©2010, Greenbranch Publishing), and *Physician Entrepreneurs: Strength in Numbers–Consolidation and Collaboration Strategies to Grow Your Practice* (©2008, HealthLeaders Media). His most recent publication is *The Healthcare Executive's Guide to ACO Strategies* (©2012, HealthLeaders Media).

A graduate of Harding University, Reiboldt is a licensed certified public accountant in Georgia and Louisiana, and a member of the American Institute of Certified Public Accountants, Healthcare Financial Management Association, and American Society of Appraisers.

About the Contributors

Aimee Greeter, MP, manager

As an integral part of Coker's financial services service line, Aimee Greeter works on a variety of consulting projects, including financial consulting, hospital accounts, practice management initiatives, as well as research and writing for various client projects. Greeter holds a Master of Public Health in Health Policy and Management from the Rollins School of Public Health at Emory University. She is an honors graduate of Michigan State University, where she attained a Bachelor of Science in Human Biology.

Gary Bell, MHA, LFACHE, senior vice president

Gary Bell serves as a senior advisor to hospital and health system executives and boards of directors, as they encounter challenges and ongoing change associated with today's evolving healthcare landscape. He also works alongside Coker's Financial Advisory Services (FAS) group in providing M&A and strategic financial advisory to healthcare facilities involved with transactions and financings. Further, Bell also works with Coker's management consulting division, providing strategic guidance to the firm's hospital and health system clients on a wide range of engagements, including hospital/medical group alignment, turnarounds and restructuring, post-merger integration and general strategic counsel. Bell holds a Bachelor of Science from Emory University and a Master of Health Administration from Georgia State University.

Justin Chamblee, MAcc, CPA, senior manager

Justin Chamblee works with clients in a variety of strategic and financial areas, mainly dealing with physician compensation and hospital-physician transactions. Chamblee holds a Bachelor of Business Administration in Accounting and a Master of Accounting from Abilene Christian University. He is licensed as a CPA in the state of Texas and is a member of the American Institute of Certified Public Accountants.

Jeffery Daigrepont, senior vice president

Jeffery Daigrepont specializes in healthcare automation, strategic planning, operations, and deployment of fully integrated information systems for medical practices and hospitals. For FY09, Daigrepont chaired the Ambulatory Information Systems Steering Committee of Healthcare Information and Management Systems Society (HIMSS). In addition, as the Ambulatory Committee liaison for

FY09 to the Annual Conference Education Committee, he represented the
HIMSS Ambulatory and Ambulatory Information Steering Committee members.

Sue Hertlein, manager

Sue Hertlein works with clients across the country on numerous technology,
strategic planning, and assessment projects. Hertlein manages research for Coker
and assists in obtaining information on new situations that affect the healthcare
industry, such as healthcare reform, meaningful use/EHR incentives, accountable
care organizations (ACO), etc. She has over 25 years of experience in the healthcare industry, with a strong background in information technology (IT).

Debbie Kiehl, manager

Debbie Kiehl is a highly accomplished practice administrator and fellow of the
American College of Medical Practice Executives. With Coker, Kiehl's focus
includes physician practice assessments, revenue cycle analysis, electronic medical
record transition, staff development, physician recruitment, operations management, and rural health clinic certification and compliance. She has a proven track
record in developing relationships with colleagues, physicians, customers, and
staff at all levels, creating an environment where measurable goals and objectives
are defined and tracked to ensure organizational success.

Madiha Khan

Madiha Khan is currently doing an internship with the Coker Group while pursuing a Master of Public Health degree in Health Management at Emory University.
As an intern, she has worked with the Financial Advisory Services and Alignment

teams on various strategic planning and physician compensation projects. Upon graduating, Khan plans to pursue a career in healthcare consulting.

Rick Langosch, FHFMA, senior vice president

Rick Langosch is a seasoned healthcare veteran, with over 25 years of experience managing operations and finance in hospitals and physician practices. Langosch works on high-level projects involving all components of healthcare. Using his wide range of financial, operational, and IT responsibilities, including multi-hospital ownership and hospital senior management positions, Langosch assists clients with interim management opportunities, physician compensation reviews, financial and revenue cycle assessments, and strategic planning.

David Melloh

David Melloh chairs Lindquist & Vennum's Health Law Group, and advises healthcare providers, such as hospitals and integrated delivery systems, physician group practices, surgery centers, and dental group practices. Having assisted clients in over 30 states, Melloh has a national reputation in structuring, negotiating, and completing healthcare transactions. He has worked with providers and managed care organizations on ACOs, clinically integrated networks, and other ventures designed to share economic risk and furnish high-quality healthcare services. Melloh has been a regular presenter at American Health Lawyers Association and other national conferences and is an adjunct faculty member at the University of Minnesota School of Public Health. He received his undergraduate degree from Carleton College, a Master of Arts from the University of Minnesota, and his law degree from Vanderbilt University School of Law, where he received academic honors and was an editor of the Vanderbilt Law Review. He has been selected repeatedly as a "Super Lawyer" and in "Best Lawyers in America."

Mark Reiboldt, MSc, senior vice president

Mark Reiboldt works in Coker's Financial Services Group and Coker Capital Advisors, the firm's investment banking division, where he advises healthcare facilities through the transaction process, including due diligence, valuation and fairness opinion, and general strategic financial advisory. He received a Bachelor of Arts in Political Science from Georgia State University and a Master of Science in Financial Economics from the University of London. Mark is a FINRA-registered securities dealer with Series 7, 63, 65, and 79 licenses.

About Coker Group

Coker Group, a national healthcare consulting firm, helps providers achieve improved financial and operational results through sound business principles. Coker's team members are proficient, trustworthy professionals with expertise and strengths in various areas, including healthcare, technology, finance, and business knowledge. Coker works with hospitals and physicians to develop sound strategies for forming and maintaining successful alliances and relationships.

Service areas include, but are not limited to: hospital-physician alignment, ACO readiness, capital advisory, strategic financial advisory and analysis, practice management, mergers/acquisitions and due diligence, compensation, pre- and post-merger integration, strategic IT planning and review, vendor vetting, managed IT services, hospital operations, medical staff development, and executive search.

Coker Group's nationwide client base includes major health systems, hospitals, physician and specialty groups, and solo practitioners in a full spectrum of engagements. Coker has gained a reputation since 1987 for thorough, efficient, and cost-conscious work to benefit its clients both financially and operationally. The members of the firm pride themselves on their client profile of recognized and respected healthcare professionals throughout the industry. Coker Group is dedicated to helping healthcare providers face today's challenges for tomorrow's successes.

Acknowledgments

Books written by Coker Group are always touched by the many people both inside and outside our organization. This work is no exception. First, we would like to give special thanks to the contributions made by our Coker team members for their dedication to researching and drafting the content offered in this publication: Gary Bell, Justin Chamblee, Jeffery Daigrepont, Aimee Greeter, Sue Hertlein, Madiha Khan, Rick Langosch, and Mark Reiboldt. In addition to our primary author, Max Reiboldt, we thank these contributors for extending their knowledge from their many years of work in medical practices and physician networks.

In addition, we thank David Melloh, partner and chair of Health Law Group, Lindquist & Vennum, a law firm based in Minneapolis, Minn., for his excellent contributions on legal and regulatory considerations.

Kay Stanley, who has contributed to Coker's 60-plus books since Coker's publishing initiative began in the early 1990s, has served as editor along with Trish Hutcherson as project manager.

Finally, we appreciate the confidence placed in Coker Group by HealthLeaders Media to relay accurate and pertinent market information.

Introduction

Alignment is a word that most of us connect to our automobiles. I learned early in life that the front end of my car must be aligned or steering would be difficult and my tires would wear out unevenly and prematurely. Without the equipment in its proper position, the car was unlikely to perform well.

In healthcare, alignment has taken on a different meaning. As its forerunner, the oft-used term in the 1980s and 1990s was *integration*. Integration is the process of blending several parties' operations and overall strategies. Indeed, during the 80s and 90s, hospitals and physicians were integrating. However, integration was a limiting term, typically meaning parties merged operations into a single "NewCo[1]," whereas alignment does not always encompass such dramatic changes.

Alignment is the process of healthcare providers working together to combine and synchronize their operations, strategies, relations, and overall delivery of care. They strive to coordinate all their services in order to respond to the market and other changes occurring within the overall delivery system. Alignment includes many forms of integration. Although the two terms can be somewhat synonymous, alignment takes the working relationships to higher and more varied levels of affiliation.

This book will focus on the dynamics between the two major and most prominent providers of healthcare—physicians and hospitals—and their alignment. Physicians still have a significant role as they provide leadership in the delivery of clinical care. Hospitals, often as major health systems[2], also provide an important part of the overall healthcare services that are so highly regarded in the United States. Thus, physicians and hospitals/health systems have continued to work together in an unprecedented approach. Alignment models have allowed the two entities to almost become one, integrating in almost every way. Yet, with alternatives to full integration, alignment models vary, depending upon the individual needs, preferences, and overall relationships of the entities. Further, the market is driving many of the models that are coming into play. Although some alignment models presented in this book may not be the primary preference of either physicians or hospitals, the providers are compelled to adopt them due to market and competitive conditions.

In delving deeply into the subject of physician-hospital alignment in this book, we will consider key areas of the various components of the physician-hospital alignment continuum. We will explore the challenges and the benefits of physician-hospital alignment in the context of current healthcare reform legislation, looking at both current law and anticipated changes. We will examine the models and break down the strategies for health systems/hospitals' application of these models.

We will also consider alternative models from the medical practice/physician's perspective as well as the hospital/health system. These models are reviewed relative to the following:

- Compensation and other financial ramifications

- Legal and regulatory components

- Information technology/systems

- Case studies using real examples of alignment strategies

Alignment in the healthcare vernacular has tremendous ramifications and complexities, which present challenges as well as opportunities. Being a part of the U.S. healthcare delivery system at this time is one of those rare opportunities to "hold on tight" as changes and new developments occur rapidly. In this book, we will examine the dynamics of the industry in the physician-hospital alignment arena.

REFERENCES

1. NewCo is a generic name for proposed corporate spin-off, startup, or subsidiary companies before they are assigned a final name, or for proposed merged companies to distinguish the to-be-formed combined entity with an existing company involved in the merger which may have the same (or a similar) name.

2. In this book, we use the terms hospital and health system synonymously—depending upon the structure and makeup of that entity.

Overview of Alignment

In the 1990s, in anticipation of a dramatic change in the structure of reimbursement, hospitals focused on purchasing practices. The thinking was that reimbursement would become a risk-based model where large groups of populations would be managed and reimbursement would be structured on a per-member/per-month capitated rate. Primary care physicians were the intended gatekeepers in the risk-based model and the federal government was to have a greater role in the management and delivery of healthcare, with overt attempts made to move toward a semi-socialistic system. Regardless of whether the political landscape changed, the perspective even in the private sector was that there would be more risk-based contracts, requiring physicians and hospitals to be integrated in the delivery of services. The response for some providers, in extreme cases, was to establish integrated delivery systems and for others, integration was a forecasted strategy for the future.

Based on their expectations of the primary gatekeeper model, hospitals began to develop their integrated delivery system through the acquisition of physician practices. Employment of those physicians soon followed on the premise that the risk-based contracts would soon unfold.

The alignment structures in the 90s were similar to, yet different from, those of today. The differences related to the way physician-alignment agreements were structured. Mostly, alignment meant employment, with little variation. Physicians were often compensated through generous guaranteed salaries with some minor incentives tied to productivity. Non-productivity-based incentives were uncommon. And, where capitation or fixed-based revenue existed, even minor incentives for productivity were diminished. Often, practices were acquired based on the determination of fair market value (FMV[1]), which was much more liberal during that period. Hospitals paid significant dollars up front for those practices, in amounts often tied to more than tangible assets—usually goodwill.

With this structure, common reasoning would be that hospitals and physicians were truly developing a partnering attitude. This was not true; something different resulted. Hospitals failed to partner with physicians in many ways, both financially and in decision-making. There was little incentive for cost management, which was a fundamental requirement under a capitated model. In fact, physicians resented hospitals' focus on cost-cutting programs.

The structures of the deals with physicians made it difficult for hospitals to obtain any return on investment as their models were dramatically flawed. The anticipated reimbursement structure, moving to risk-based contracts and capitated income, never significantly unfolded in the private sector. Although capitation did take hold in some parts of the country and still exists to some extent, for the most part, this system of reimbursement and overall structure never prevailed. By the end of the 90s, many health systems concluded that strategically, operationally, and economically, they did not need to continue to employ physicians.

Their losses were massive, and for the most part, the physicians were not happy with their structure. Administrative management and oversight were largely inefficient and ineffective. Thus, the attempt at integration and alignment in the 90s essentially failed.

Entering the 21st century, some forms of physician-hospital integration began to resurface. Concurrently, many hospitals continued to divest their employed physicians, while others lost interest in expanding that structure. Mutually, physicians preferred to continue in private practices.

Further, physicians—particularly specialists—sought ways to augment their incomes by moving into new service areas previously considered as hospitals' "turf." Private practice physicians began to own and operate surgery centers, diagnostic clinics, sleep centers, and various ancillary services to supplement their income from professional fees and in an effort to deliver services to patients more efficiently, conveniently, and economically than by the hospital.

Essentially, the physician-hospital integration paradigm largely disappeared in many areas. Physicians fundamentally preferred being in private practice.

Meanwhile, fee-for-service was the primary reimbursement structure across private, state, and federal payer programs. The stresses on the healthcare delivery system continued to increase from virtually all perspectives, as the first decade of the 21st century ended. The cost of delivery continued to escalate well above inflation rates, for example. Today, achieving reimbursement from third-party payers and the government at existing fee-for-service rates is increasingly challenged. Also, some physicians have an unrelenting desire to order extensive tests and services (not discouraged in a fee-for-service environment), which continue to drive up utilization, costs, and the overall amounts spent on healthcare.

Private and government payers finally have realized that fee-for-service is an unsustainable model, as evidenced by the passage of the Patient Protection and Affordable Care Act healthcare reform in March 2010. Without debating the pros and cons of that particular law, this legislation represents an attempt by the federal government to place constraints on healthcare providers. Private insurers are also moving in this direction at a rapid pace. This is largely fueled by the stresses on the system of increased costs, higher utilization, and the socioeconomic strain in our country, which includes an aging population, an increasing number of foreign-born individuals entering the United States, and a growing number of uninsured patients.

The outcome is this: physician-hospital alignment is once again rising in importance in order to meet the challenges of the times. Hospitals, by necessity, are purchasing practices, but at FMV tangible asset value, which entails little up-front payments and virtually no goodwill. Reimbursement remains primarily as fee-for-service, though incentives for cost controls, quality outcomes, and patient satisfaction (i.e., something other than direct physician productivity) is under discussion. Nevertheless, physician productivity is still the key matrix in the provider compensation structures under the employment model (or models similar to employment) through a professional services agreement (PSA).

As hospitals and physicians are integrating again, they are now truly looking at alignment, which may not always connote employment. Moreover, they are looking for ways to form true partnerships that focus on quality of patient care, delivery of services, and cost-effective management. As noted, non-employment models that range from simply working together on a limited contractual basis to full forms of alignment (but actually not including employment) are now considered in the continuum of this process.

Hospitals/health systems have come a long way toward realizing a value proposition in alignment. Many of them acquire the ancillaries developed by the private practice physician groups, paying at FMV rates, and capturing the revenue stream going forward. For now, the federal government, through the Medicare and Medicaid system, often pays more to hospitals that bill for those same ancillary services under a hospital outpatient department structure.

Most hospitals today are adopting a broader approach to physician-hospital alignment. They understand that they need to work closely with their physicians, but the relationship is not limited to an employment model, particularly like those structured in the past. More emphasis is now placed on information technology (IT) and clinical integration where continuity of care is a primary goal. Communication and the exchange of information data that is essential to managing cost and realizing greater quality outcomes is dependent upon clinical integration.

Physicians' Interest in Aligning With Hospitals

There are a number of reasons physicians are interested in aligning with hospitals, but the primary reasons include:

- Financial stability through improved compensation

- Shared risk

- Improved quality of life

- Infrastructure support to off-load administrative duties

- Practice style (shift variances to hospital)

- Recruitment and retention (private practices cannot compete with hospitals)

- Succession strategy (no cash-out value in private practices)

Financial stability is a challenge for physicians; therefore, they are looking to hospitals to partner with and to achieve improved compensation. Beyond employment, alignment arrangements may be through a PSA or some other limited services contract that allows the physicians to be compensated for the work that they do and for the hospitals to improve their return on investment. All such compensation must be at FMV and commercially reasonable rates, as defined in Chapter 9. Arrangements must be made within specific guidelines, with each particular plan measured within its individual and specific tenets.

Another reason for physicians to align with hospitals is the ever-increasing risk of malpractice liability and the cost of the insurance protection from lawsuits. Although malpractice insurance costs have somewhat stabilized in comparison to earlier years, it remains a major factor for physicians to partner with hospitals to share the risk in liability. Often, larger health systems have a self-insurance plan that effectively lowers the cost of the malpractice insurance by spreading the expenditure over a larger pool of physicians.

Lifestyle is another reason that many physicians want to align with hospitals. Although not new, quality of life issues seem to be more central, especially among younger physicians just coming out of training. Although they are as dedicated to their careers and the clinical quality of their practice as older physicians, newer physicians are less concerned about practice ownership and being devoted to that business. Rather, many want someone else (e.g., a hospital or corporate entity) to provide the administrative and management services, so that they can commit professional time to clinical services. Certainly, some physicians want control and active involvement in their businesses; however, fewer physicians are interested in working additional hours in order to manage the business.

Although hospitals did a rather poor job of managing practices in the 90s, the infrastructure support that they can provide today is much better. This includes one of the top reasons for many physicians to align with hospitals in the context of infrastructure support—the hospital's ability to provide advanced IT support. This is a key point that must be considered going forward. There is no alternative to a medical practice having an electronic health record and related IT support. Chapter 11 explores the IT arena in the context of physician-hospital alignment.

Shifting practice style variances to the hospital is another reason for many physicians to become aligned. The means letting the hospital partner with the practice in developing the full continuum of services and balancing the differing practice styles under an alignment structure. As often seen in larger single- and multi-specialty groups, physicians differ in practice styles; these variances are best dealt with within a hospital infrastructure.

Physician recruitment and retention is another challenge best handled by health systems. Private practices are under continual stress for adding new providers to increase revenue. Many private practices within particular specialties simply cannot compete with the local and regional market requirements, such as compensation and benefits including income guarantees, tuition payments, etc. (The recruitment/incubation alignment strategy is discussed in Chapter 4.) As hospitals are better equipped to meet market demands in these areas, it makes good sense for practices to shift physician recruitment and retention to hospitals.

Finally, many private practices are struggling with their existing buy-in/buy-out terms and conditions. Often, these terms were set so that departing physicians were required to be "cashed out"; now, liquid funds are not available in private practices. Younger physicians coming into the partnership or practices are not interested in a large buy-in amount, which again challenges the very existence of the private practice. Developing a mechanism where succession planning works within the hospital alignment structure is becoming of interest to physicians.

Hospitals' Interest in Aligning With Physicians

The main reasons hospitals are looking to align with physicians include:

- Market share

    – Recruitment and retention

- Accountable care

- Response to physicians' needs

  – Administrative

  – Financial

- Long-term sustainability

Hospitals and health systems are understandably concerned about maintaining a share of the market so that they can remain viable. Being able to capture a base of physicians—from primary care to specialists—through alignment is the foundation for maintaining market share.

Aligning with physicians also helps ensure success in both recruitment and retention efforts. Recruitment is a major challenge; however, this challenge can be reduced when physicians know they have an option as to various alignment models. Likewise, retention is a major part of any hospital's strategy relative to its medical staff. Being able to retain physicians because of the varied alignment strategy is a major benefit. Again, the broader approach to alignment helps because it gives physicians more independence.

Moving into the era of accountable care, hospitals and health systems must have a full pool of physicians that will be a part of their accountable care organization (ACO). Although ACOs do not require physicians to be employed (they can be contracted by the ACO), the ability to recruit and retain physicians will be largely dependent upon the level of alignment that exists. This is particularly the case with primary care, as the Medicare ACO requires that primary care physicians only become a part of one ACO instead of several at one time.

Responding to physicians' needs has long been a reason for hospitals to align with their medical staffs. As mentioned at the beginning of this chapter, this was a major thrust of the employment model of the 90s—and still is. But it also can be effectuated through other forms of alignment, which we will discuss in more detail throughout the book. Hospitals are responding to both administrative and financial needs of physicians. Administratively, physicians often are frustrated and weary of the day-to-day hassles and responsibilities of managing and operating the non-clinical portion of their practice (i.e., the business side). And financially, many physicians' incomes have been cut by reduced reimbursement and escalating costs. The ability for hospitals to respond to physicians' financial and administrative needs, while still maintaining FMV and commercially reasonable compensation rates, is a major reason hospitals are aligning with their medical staff.

As also discussed earlier in this chapter, hospitals and physicians have struggled over the years with trust and good relationships with each other. Now, hospitals are seeking ways to align to improve relations with individual physicians. Working through various alignment models is a viable goal and objective relative to hospitals' alignment strategies.

Finally, long-term sustainability is a major goal for hospitals in their alignment strategy. Hospitals provide services within the healthcare continuum that cannot be fulfilled by other entities, but they must have physicians in order to offer these services. Thus, to realize such long-term sustainability, it is essential to have loyal and aligned physicians in the healthcare system.

Current Trends

We must understand that current trends are similar to the experiences in the early 1990s. For example, a recent survey[2] stated that 81% of hospital leaders indicated a moderate to high interest in acquiring practices/engaging physicians in employment. They also acknowledged that types of alignment other than employment are under way and of interest. Thus, a key trend today is stronger collaboration between hospitals and health systems and physicians and practices.

Figure 1.1 illustrates that specifically, relative to government forms of reimbursements, health systems and practices are responding through greater forms of

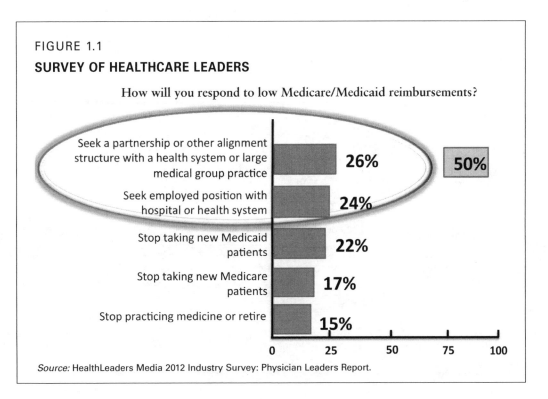

FIGURE 1.1

SURVEY OF HEALTHCARE LEADERS

How will you respond to low Medicare/Medicaid reimbursements?

Seek a partnership or other alignment structure with a health system or large medical group practice — 26% — **50%**

Seek employed position with hospital or health system — 24%

Stop taking new Medicaid patients — 22%

Stop taking new Medicare patients — 17%

Stop practicing medicine or retire — 15%

Source: HealthLeaders Media 2012 Industry Survey: Physician Leaders Report.

alignment. Statistics from Merritt Hawkins' 2012 report of its recruiting assignments indicate that 63% of physician recruitment in 2011 was for hospitals—up
from 56% the previous year and only 11% as recent as eight years ago. Moreover,
family physicians and general internists top the list of the most common physician
recruitment assignments. This illustrates that hospitals are becoming the choice of
full alignment, often through employment of physicians. The Merritt Hawkins
report concludes that three of four physicians hired in the year 2014 will work for
a hospital.

Figure 1.2 illustrates a survey from a HealthLeaders Media Intelligence Report
wherein the question was asked: Which of the following physician specialties are
most relevant to your organization's M&A strategy? Primary care was at the
forefront; but interestingly, some of the "higher-end" specialties such as orthopedics, cardiology, and others are also ranked very high at or above 50% of
their strategy.

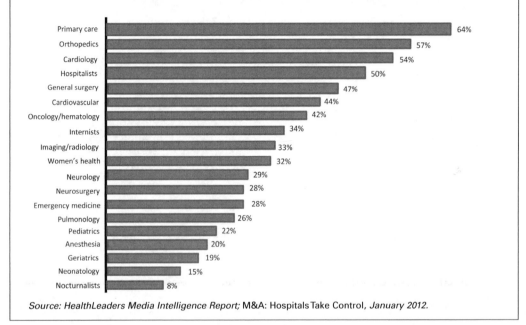

FIGURE 1.2

SURVEY OF HEALTHCARE LEADERS

Q. Which of the following physician specialties are most relevant to your organization's M&A strategy?

Specialty	Percentage
Primary care	64%
Orthopedics	57%
Cardiology	54%
Hospitalists	50%
General surgery	47%
Cardiovascular	44%
Oncology/hematology	42%
Internists	34%
Imaging/radiology	33%
Women's health	32%
Neurology	29%
Neurosurgery	28%
Emergency medicine	28%
Pulmonology	26%
Pediatrics	22%
Anesthesia	20%
Geriatrics	19%
Neonatology	15%
Nocturnalists	8%

Source: HealthLeaders Media Intelligence Report; M&A: Hospitals Take Control, *January 2012.*

Summary

Alignment strategies are in place and are being considered by virtually every physician and hospital in the United States. Physicians and hospitals both face unprecedented challenges in their ability to maintain viability. Partnering alternatives are, without question, the best solution for responding to these challenging issues, such as new federal and state structures, ACOs, and the like. Hospitals and physicians should assume a broad approach to alignment, not necessarily a "one-size-fits-all" approach. Employment or employment "lite" models are not always the models of choice. Therefore, it is necessary to consider options and alternatives and be responsive to each individual situation.

It is also important to keep in mind the key alignment challenges. These include:

- Culture

- Operations

- Autonomy and control

- Trust

- Competition

- Sharing revenue

Discussed in more detail throughout this book, these key points must be addressed within every relationship between hospital and physician leaders. Each point must be a part of the overall deal because they are all important parts of the entire physician-hospital alignment structure.

REFERENCES

1. The IRS defines fair market value as the price at which property or the right to use property would change hands between a willing buyer and a willing seller, neither being under an compulsion to buy, sell, or transfer property or the right to use property, and both having reasonable knowledge of the facts.

2. HealthLeaders Media-Intelligence; *M&A: Hospitals Take Control,* January 2012.

2

Strength in Numbers and Other Alignment Benefits

Alignment in healthcare today occurs for multiple reasons, as discussed in Chapter 1. One important outcome realized through alignment is "strength in numbers." The strength in numbers concept is familiar to most people, as it applies to a number of industries, not just healthcare. For example, auto industry unions, such as the United Auto Workers (UAW), are an example of strength in numbers throughout the history of America's auto industry. Through the UAW, auto industry workers (along with those in other industries represented by UAW) have achieved labor and compensation standards that may not have been achieved without the ability to collectively bargain with employers. The basis for the strength in numbers concept is that people working together for a central purpose are more likely to succeed than those who face work challenges alone. In this chapter, we discuss ways that the strength in numbers concept applies within healthcare—specifically in aligned relationships—and proffers advantages to health systems, physicians, and patients.

Strength in Numbers' Impact on Health Systems

One of the reasons health systems want to align with physicians is to increase the size and strength of their overall provider network. For example, many health systems are interested in aligning with primary care physicians, who will then "feed" the remainder of the specialty physicians within the health system. This type of thinking reinforces that the health system, while made up of individual and multiple parts, relies on all of these parts as a whole to be successful. Once the health system aligns with primary care physicians who are dedicated to seeing the system succeed, it has found a way to ensure other segments of the system (namely, the specialists) are more likely to be successful as well. In this way, most systems realize that to be successful, they need to have a greater number of primary care physicians who can support their key growth and development goals.

Building upon the strength in numbers concept, health systems also recognize that aligning with primary care physicians reduces competition. For example, when Health System A acquires a primary care practice and employs its physicians, it eliminates the possibility for Health System B to do the same; this results in a stronger physician network for Health System A, and proactively stymies additional competition from Health System B.

Another way that strength in numbers applies to aligned relationships is that when health systems work collaboratively with their physicians, they are able to ensure a wider scope of services is offered. Most hospitals are utilizing a multiple approach to alignment, meaning that they are pursuing alignment through various structural models and with different groups and specialties. This is often a wise strategic decision on the part of the system, as alignment is typically not best effected through a "one-size-fits-all" approach. As a result, health systems are beginning to appreciate the fact that they can extend their reach further once they align with a wider expanse of physicians and specialties. Often, the ability to provide a greater scope of services bolsters the hospital's reputation in the market and can help retain patients who want to receive all of their services in one place. In short, being able to offer a comprehensive range of services, as is possible through an alignment strategy, helps the hospital better meet a community's needs.

While health systems have historically been competitors with physicians, the popularity of alignment has allowed health systems to realize that they become stronger when they *work* with, as opposed to *compete* with, their medical staff.

Strength in Numbers' Impact on Physicians

Today, the pressures on private practice physicians are greater than they perhaps have ever been. Declining reimbursement, increased supply expenses, competition from other practices and hospitals, and a necessity to actively manage the medical practice in addition to a busy clinical practice are just a few examples. Through alignment, however, many of these pressures are reduced or eliminated. Therefore, one of the most significant effects of alignment on physicians is the ability to shift some of the pressures they currently face to their strategic partner.

Contracting with private payers is one example of a key pressure facing physicians today. In a time when physicians feel additional recognition is warranted for the medical services they perform, payers are cutting back on reimbursement. Although many practices are able to achieve rates from private payers that are equal to 110% or greater of the Medicare fee schedule, there are other practices that are forced, by virtue of the market in which they operate, to accept reimbursement at or below Medicare rates. When practices align with a health system and transition the responsibility for payer contracting to that system, almost without exception the rates practices receive going forward are greater than what they had received historically. This is because they gain strength in aligning with a system that negotiates on their behalf as part of the larger entity. Although the increase in reimbursement from payers varies by specialty and certainly by market, health systems typically receive 5%–15% greater reimbursement than the physician practices in their same community.

In many alignment models, practices are able to enjoy the benefit of these greater reimbursement rates. While the increased reimbursement cannot be shared directly with physicians for compliance reasons, the higher total revenue increases the pool of funds available for distribution to physicians as compensation. As a result, physicians may experience higher compensation than they had historically because of improved payer contracts. This, however, is only possible because they were able to leverage strength in numbers by aligning with a health system.

Another key pressure faced by physicians today is increasing competition from hospitals. Physicians and hospitals have always been competitors, but many physicians feel this pressure has increased in recent years. In fact, alignment can be seen as a driver for this increase in competition. As many hospitals begin to employ greater numbers of their medical staff, other physicians see themselves as being "shut out" and feel that the employed physicians are given preferential marketing, easier access to block time, and other perks not afforded to private practice physicians that make it easier for the employed physicians to be successful. One way to face the increasing pressures from other physicians and their health system partners is to become aligned as well. Think of the old adage, "If you can't beat 'em, join 'em." Once aligned, physicians are part of a supportive network in which to succeed, rather than being seen as a competitor. Now the aligned physicians may become privy to increased marketing efforts on their behalf, more operating room time, and the like, which allows them to better compete with other physician groups. Strength in numbers is on their side. Physicians can effectively mitigate the number of challenges they face today through partnering. Alignment allows them to share responsibility with another entity, often one that is larger in size and stature, and can help bear the burdens of the day-to-day practice.

Strength in Numbers' Impact on Patients

Some communities fear that consolidation between hospitals and physicians will result in the rationing of care for patients under the guise of more streamlined, cost-effective care. Largely, this is because patients have a limited understanding of what alignment means, and what hospitals and physicians seek to achieve as a result of it. They may not understand that *lower-cost* care at the risk of *lower-quality* care would never be in a hospital's best interests (or physicians or patients). Moreover, patients may potentially have the most to gain as a result of alignment.

As opposed to lower-quality care or fewer services, patients stand to benefit significantly from alignment. One benefit is the transparency of data that can result. Often, when physicians and hospitals align, they transition to a common information technology (IT) platform; most often, physicians adopt the inpatient and ambulatory IT systems within the health system. This allows patients nearly seamless care across a host of providers. For example, through the physician and hospital's interconnected IT system, physicians are able to access lab results, imaging tests, and orders for a patient made by another physician. Having access to a wealth of historical and concurrent data from other providers allows physicians to best treat their patients. It can help reduce the risk of prescription drug interactions, duplicative testing, and overlapping care. This level of IT integration would be more challenging—and maybe not possible—without alignment.

In addition, many organizations now offer the ability for patients to access their medical records through a Web-based portal. In this single portal, a patient can log in to the website using his or her secure user name and password and access medical records and test results, schedule appointments at both physician offices and the hospital, and communicate with a wide range of providers, who can also view this same information for their common patients. Through a connected communication network and shared data channels made possible by common IT, patients also benefit from strength in numbers.

In review, alignment allows health systems and physicians to join forces and leverage their shared strengths. Their strength in numbers results in improvements for health systems, physicians, and patients.

Overarching Pros and Cons of Alignment

Chapter 1 outlined many of the reasons alignment is currently being pursued by hospitals and physicians alike. In this chapter, we identify several of the overarching pros and cons of alignment. The advantages currently being experienced may be offset by the factor that they are not guaranteed for the future.

Economics

Many physicians see alignment with a health system as a way to increase (or at least stabilize) their compensation. One pervasive real-life example of this is cardiology. Due to the Medicare reimbursement cuts implemented in 2008, private practice cardiologists realized a significant decline in reimbursement for their nuclear and echocardiogram studies. Overnight, the same procedures rendered in the same location by the same technicians and interpreted by the same physicians were reimbursed by Medicare at 80% or less of the prior-year reimbursement. These services, which had historically had a tremendous profit margin, were beginning to run at a loss in some practices. As a result, many cardiologists began to look at alignment with a health system to eliminate further erosion of their income.

At present, hospitals are still able to pursue reimbursement methodologies for Medicare patients that are not availed to physicians, such as hospital outpatient department (HOPD) rates and provider-based billing (PBB). In the case of cardiology, many practices sell (or lease) their nuclear and echo machines to their local hospital, which can take advantage of HOPD rates. In this manner, hospitals are able to receive significantly greater reimbursement for the same ancillary cardiology tests, even when they are offered in the physician's practice. It is important to note that HOPD billing for ancillaries requires a number of criteria be met, including mileage restrictions, appropriate signage, a separate entrance, etc. As part of the due diligence process, health systems need to ensure they meet all criteria before they begin billing as an HOPD.

In addition, hospitals can pursue PBB for aligned physicians, which allows for greater reimbursement for ambulatory services (primarily evaluation and management services). The magnitude of the increase under PBB reimbursement may be less than the increase for services billed as an HOPD; however, it is still greater than the amount the practice is eligible to receive. In a time when every penny counts for healthcare organizations, HOPD and PBB are an attractive reimbursement methodology. While no one is certain how long these types of payments will last (as many do not consider this methodology to make sound fiscal sense in that the same procedures would be paid at such different rates), they are a viable, compliant strategy at present.

As a result of their ability to participate in alternative reimbursement methodologies which afford them greater revenue, hospitals are in a position to share this increased revenue with physicians (although, as noted earlier in the chapter, this cannot be shared directly, particularly for Medicare patients). In turn, the physicians realize greater compensation than they had historically. Therefore, a compelling economic return for both health systems and physicians is one of the overarching pros of alignment.

Operations

In a market that has multiple hospitals within a single health system in a limited geographic area, many practices provide services at multiple organizations. This is often seen in a large metropolitan area where a health system has a single large hospital, as well as smaller hospitals in the suburbs or nearby outlying areas. While this may be necessary due to the complexity of services to be provided (for example, Hospital A may have the appropriate equipment and technology to support pediatric orthopedic procedures, while Hospital B may not; as a result, all pediatric orthopedic cases within a specific orthopedic practice are taken to Hospital A), in many cases the need for practices to perform services at multiple hospitals decreases their operational efficiency. However, in an aligned relationship, there is often the opportunity to realize more streamlined operations.

In the example above, Hospital A may be willing to assign block scheduling for pediatric orthopedic cases, thereby guaranteeing physicians dedicated operating room time to complete their cases. Or, the health system may be willing to hire a mid-level provider who would support the orthopedists (both in the operating room and by rounding on inpatients) so they can be more efficient. Also, the system may be willing to provide economic support (through a guaranteed salary or payment for windshield time[1]) to the orthopedists so there is not a punitive impact to the physicians as a result of their coverage of multiple systems.

One of the overarching pros for alignment is the ability for physicians and health systems to work together to improve operational efficiencies and to do so in a way that will increase revenue for the system and protect the income of the physicians.

Data sharing

While fee-for-service has historically been the driver for payment within the healthcare industry, in an accountable care world, it is likely that the primary drivers will be focused on quality and outcomes. To demonstrate high-quality and positive outcomes, all organizations must look closely at their IT systems. Organizations that are unable to track quality and outcomes will be unable to report on them; in turn, they may find themselves in a situation where they will not be paid for services. However, implementing IT can be costly, and widespread data sharing cannot occur without multiple parties contributing information into the system. Hospitals are often willing to bear the costs of implementing IT for their aligned physicians, recognizing the potential down-stream (i.e., future) dividends it may provide. Likewise, physicians are more willing to actively participate in a common IT system post-alignment with its strategic partner and find direct value in this shared reporting. With a shared vision in mind, developing comprehensive data sharing between hospitals and physicians becomes much easier in an aligned relationship. And this data sharing will improve quality and outcomes, which may ultimately drive reimbursement.

While a change to reimbursement based on quality and outcomes may still be on the horizon, it is more likely to occur than ever before. Participation in a comprehensive IT system that allows for shared data, as is made possible under an aligned model, becomes a proactive way for health systems and physicians to prepare for the future.

Responsiveness in an accountable care era

As discussed earlier in this chapter (and in further detail in Chapter 3), one of the overarching pros of alignment is the opportunity it provides both physicians and hospitals to work more closely together in an effort to adapt to the changing reimbursement paradigm and the new accountable care era in which we find ourselves today. Having an alignment structure in place becomes the foundation upon which accountable care structures can then be built, whether it is a patient-centered medical home, a clinically integrated network, a quality collaborative, or an accountable care organization. Just as alignment does not need to mean employment, accountable care structures also do not require employment to be at the foundation of their model. Many of the new accountable care structures work well with non-employment, contractual relationships.

Cons of alignment

Although alignment has a number of positive attributes, there are also some potential challenges associated with it. One of the most significant is the pervasive lack of trust that can be inherent in these relationships. Physicians often feel that they have lost some control over the practice, which creates discomfort and potentially some friction with the hospital. Some hospitals also prefer to oversee and unduly control the practices with which they have aligned, thereby creating a legitimate loss of autonomy for the physicians.

In some of the more complex forms of alignment, there are longer-term contracts that tie the parties together, which can make an unwind more difficult. Unwinding the arrangement (through the necessary legal or financial steps) can also be a challenge in models where assets are purchased and would need to repurchased by the original party.

Physicians also struggle with the fact that non-compete clauses are often present in their agreements with the hospital, which can make separation difficult, particularly in cases where the non-compete allows them to return only to private practice (but not align with another hospital/health system for a defined period of time).

Finally, sometimes alignment relationships can become burdened with bureaucracy, causing decisions about the practice, including staffing, to be slow moving. Physicians in private practice are typically able to be quite nimble, and as a result do not understand or agree with the time it may take to get decisions made and implemented.

Summary

Like many industries, healthcare has found a way to utilize the strength in numbers concept to create the greatest possible outcomes. Overall, it has resulted in positive change for health systems, physicians, and patients. In a way never seen before, alignment is helping different components of the healthcare continuum come together in support of common goals: patient-centered care, improved quality, and positive outcomes.

REFERENCE

1. Unproductive work-related time spent in the car is known as "windshield time."

Healthcare Reform and Related Structures

Healthcare reform, effectuated through governmental regulation and legislation, is impacting the status of the healthcare environment significantly. In fact, health-care reform is the primary driver of changing delivery models and is still being vetted within political, legal (via the highest courts in the land), and legislative circles at both the federal and state levels. Where this will all take us is still an unanswered question. Will we continue with a mostly private healthcare delivery system? Will the government have a greater role? Will we ultimately go to a single payer system? Are we headed toward a socialized system similar to Great Britain, France, Canada, and other countries? Will reimbursement from private and governmental payers be bundled into essentially one payment for the providers to share/divide? Will we vacate a mostly fee-for-service reimbursement prototype for a fee-for-value system?

These and other questions must and will be answered soon. Their answers will affect the physician-hospital alignment structures, timing, economic relations—indeed, the entire healthcare environment. This chapter addresses many of these new thoughts and formats in the context of healthcare reform.

Accountable Care Organizations

Accountable care organizations (ACO) and the Centers for Medicare & Medicaid Services' (CMS) Electronic Health Records (EHR) Incentive Programs are probably the two most discussed items in today's healthcare arena. Accountable care is and will continue to be a major focus for most healthcare providers. Various forms of ACOs have existed for several years, with the launch of formal CMS ACOs occurring January 1, 2012. Currently, there are CMS ACOs, private (commercial) ACOs, and providers offering accountable care outside of formal organizations. Such entities are often formed through clinically integrated networks (CIN) and/or quality collaboratives (QC). They look like and have many of the features of ACOs, and are sometimes referred to as "ACO lite." These models offer physicians and hospitals financial incentives to provide quality care to patients, while reducing and maintaining costs. These entities (CINs, QCs, ACOs) hold participating providers jointly accountable for patient care and outcomes, and as a result, require the providers to work in a highly collaborative environment. Alignments for physician to physician, physician to hospital, and to other providers are essential to the success of any ACO entity. Physicians and hospitals must trust each other and work together to provide patient-centered quality care, while reducing costs.

Many private ACOs are sponsored by large employers that have a vested interest in having a healthier community and reducing claim costs. Typically, these are self-funded employers that bear most of the financial responsibility for health claims, with a reinsurance policy to protect them from an extremely large single claim or substantial aggregate claims. The local healthcare providers know how important it is to have the corporations' employees as their patients; thus, they participate in the employers' plans. When such large companies require the formation of some type of accountable care model to improve the quality of care and health of their employees—while reducing claim costs—they, in essence, force the providers to form some sort of alliance (i.e., alignment) to meet these requirements. The providers must work in tandem to ensure excellent communications and appropriate treatment plans for the patients they share.

The primary focus of the CMS ACOs, as well as many of the private ones, is to reduce or eliminate hospital stays, reduce emergency room visits, and better manage chronic care. The higher costs are typically related to hospitalizations and chronic care, which is a part of the reason why Medicare claims continue to grow at accelerated rates. Figure 3.1 illustrates a projected increase in Medicare benefits of 29% from 2011 to 2015.

According to a study conducted by the National Center for Health Statistics, the average length of stay (LOS) for hospitalizations in 2011 for all ages was 4.9 days. For patients 65–74 years old, the average LOS was 5.5 days, and the average LOS was 5.8 days for patients 75–84 years of age[1]. Typically, as patients grow older, their hospital LOS increases. One focus of Medicare ACOs is reducing patients' LOS as well as reducing new admissions and readmissions. A common issue for Medicare beneficiaries is seeing multiple physicians and then having to remember physicians' instructions, medication dosage, etc., from all of them. Developing strong provider collaborations through various ACO alignments will help reduce the redundancy of tests and the risk of medication contradictions, improve quality of care, and result in healthier patients and reduced claim costs.

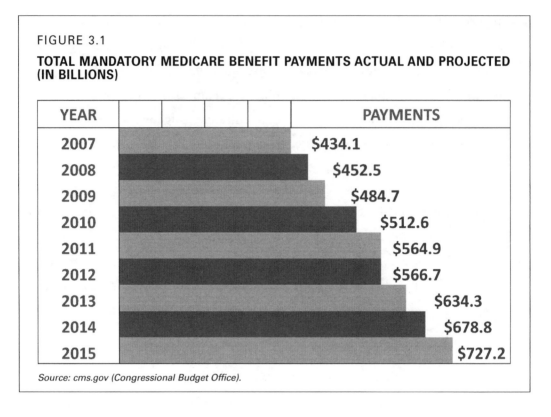

FIGURE 3.1

TOTAL MANDATORY MEDICARE BENEFIT PAYMENTS ACTUAL AND PROJECTED (IN BILLIONS)

YEAR					PAYMENTS
2007					$434.1
2008					$452.5
2009					$484.7
2010					$512.6
2011					$564.9
2012					$566.7
2013					$634.3
2014					$678.8
2015					$727.2

Source: cms.gov (Congressional Budget Office).

The potential for forming some type of ACO in a community in the future has increased physician-hospital alignment and further developed the need for collaboration now. In some of the CMS ACO models, the providers must share in any savings, as well as losses. Clinical integration is at the core of the ACO and ACO lite models. As discussed in detail in Chapter 11, this encourages the development of integrated technology to collect, report, and analyze data to meet all goals. It also necessitates the establishment of frequent communications between all providers to safeguard the outcomes of both quality of care and costs.

Patient-Centered Medical Homes

Patient-centered medical homes (PCMH), like ACOs, are rising in prominence. PCMHs took a back seat to the accountable care world, which was the focus of 2011 and 2012. Now, thousands of PCMHs exist. However, you may be unfamiliar with exactly what PCMHs are and what role they play. The National Committee for Quality Assurance (NCQA[2]) defines a PCMH as follows:

The Patient Centered Medical Home is a health care setting that facilitates partnerships between individual patients, and their personal physicians, and when appropriate, the patient's family or caregivers. Care is facilitated by registries, information technology, health information exchange and other means to ensure that patients get the indicated care when and where they need and want it in a culturally and linguistically appropriate manner.

PCMH principles include:

- Strong primary care physician-patient relationship

- Improved access (24/7) to physician or qualified provider

- Quality and safety

- Continuity of care and coordination of care

- Holistic care (whole person)

The NCQA initiated a certification program in 2011 that identified elements that must be met in six categories. Those categories are:

1. Enhance access and continuity of care

2. Identify and manage patient populations

3. Plan and manage care

4. Provide self-care support and community resources

5. Track and coordinate care

6. Measure and improve performance

A typical structure for a PCMH requires the patient's primary care physician (PCP) to be the first contact for all care, which is often supplemented by a care coordinator. The PCP leads a team of other healthcare professionals in the delivery of care to the patient in an ambulatory setting. The other providers could include home healthcare professionals (e.g., nurses, therapists, nutritional counselors, medical equipment suppliers), ambulatory providers (e.g., dialysis centers, physical therapy centers, pharmacies), and other physicians (e.g., cardiologists, nephrologists, oncologists) based upon the patient's diagnosis. When the patient requires acute care, a hospital then becomes part of the team for an interim period.

Some PCPs have started their own initiatives to create a PCMH environment; and in some communities, medium-to-large employers are sponsoring PCMH programs as they recognize the importance of these types of models. Many of the established ACOs throughout the country combine the elements, if not the actual structure, of a PCMH in their model. After all, two of the main focal points of the ACO are patient-centered care and reducing costs. The PCMH philosophy is completely patient-focused and also reduces costs by treating the patient holistically in an ambulatory environment, most frequently in the patient's home. Because the PCMH is easier and less costly to form, it is currently a more prominent healthcare concept than ACOs. But clearly, PCMHs form the foundation of an ACO or accountable care-type model, especially if the current Medicare ACO model changes prior to complete implementation and application.

The PCMH model requires full collaboration between providers, with the patient's PCP at the helm of the ship. It does not necessarily require a formal alignment, but it does require the providers to work in tandem to support the patient and provide the best care possible. Thus, PCMHs are a viable alternative (for now) to ACOs, though PCMHs will not replace ACOs. Like the ACOs, PCMHs no longer allow providers to practice in a silo; providers must work together as a team to form a partnership with the patient's best interest as their focus. The PCMH structure also requires the patient and caregivers to partner with the healthcare providers and take more responsibility for decisions regarding the patient's care, the administration and compliance of care and, ultimately, the outcomes. Overall, the PCMH is a viable, first-step strategy, whereas the ACO is a more costly and uncertain approach to a not-fully-vetted changing reimbursement paradigm. However, both entities complement a physician-hospital alignment strategy.

American Recovery and Reinvestment Act

Congress passed the American Recovery and Reinvestment Act of 2009 (ARRA) at the urging of President Barack Obama as a direct response to the economic crisis of that time. The Recovery Act had three immediate goals:

- Create new jobs and save existing ones

- Spur economic activity and invest in long-term growth

- Foster unprecedented levels of accountability and transparency in government spending

ARRA intended to achieve those goals by providing $787 billion for tax cuts and benefits for millions of working families and businesses; funding for entitlement programs, such as unemployment benefits; and funding for federal contracts, grants, and loans. Now a few years after this act was passed and the injection of these billions of dollars, virtually all of which were funded with borrowed money by the federal government—thus contributing to the federal deficit—the U.S. economy has not responded. While the healthcare industry continues to be vibrant, the issues of controlling costs have largely not yet been addressed. Hence, the emphasis on physician-hospital alignment, accountable care, clinical integration, and technology advancement are viable and necessary.

ARRA funding

Although there are various aspects of ARRA that affect healthcare, this section only addresses those with a direct (or indirect) link to alignment. Under the federal grants portion of ARRA, the Health Information Technology for Economic and Clinical Health Act was introduced into law. One aspect of the law was to stimulate automation adoption in healthcare, known as the CMS EHR Incentive Programs. This is probably the most well-known healthcare provision of ARRA. (Some incorrectly believe that the EHR incentive program was part of the Patient Protection and Affordable Care Act, when it is actually funded under ARRA.) This incentive program provides funding to qualified healthcare professionals and hospitals that meaningfully use a certified electronic system for patient records. The plan actually has two programs: one falls under Medicare and the other is under state-managed Medicaid. Under the Medicare program, eligible providers and hospitals who fail to implement and properly utilize an EHR will have their Medicare reimbursements reduced beginning in 2015. (There are no penalties under the Medicaid program.) As of July 2012, the federal government had paid out over $6.5 billion to eligible healthcare professionals and hospitals under the CMS EHR Incentive Programs for the meaningful use of electronic health technology.

In some instances, physician practices have joined together to increase their vendor purchasing power for an EHR system. Greater numbers of physicians buying a system can translate into a greater vendor discount on an EHR package. Additionally, some hospitals have purchased technology systems for their acute care needs that also contain an ambulatory solution for practices. Some of these hospitals are offering the ambulatory EHRs at a discounted rate to their community physicians. The hospitals can include a further discount with the relaxation of the Stark Law.[3] When hospitals, physicians, and medical groups share the same basic EHR system, it allows them to easily share patient data, while still protecting confidential financial data for each provider.

Under ARRA, the U.S. Department of Health and Human Services Office of the National Coordinator for Health Information Technology awarded millions in grants to establish 60 Health Information Technology Regional Extension Centers (REC) across the country. The RECs are intended to provide a local resource for technical assistance, guidance, and information on best practices in implementing EHRs for primary care providers, critical access hospitals, and rural hospitals. The RECs are directly related to the CMS EHR Incentive Programs, since they provide funding to assist PCPs and other certain eligible providers with the selection and implementation of a certified system.

Another provision of the ARRA law encourages the development and expansion of Health Information Exchanges (HIE) at a state level. Actually, HIE is a term used to describe both the sharing of health information electronically among two or more entities, and it also refers to an organization which provides services that enable the electronic sharing of health information. The increased availability of relevant health information through HIE[4]:

- Provides a key building block for improved patient care, quality, and safety

- Makes relevant healthcare information available where and when it is needed

- Provides the connecting point for an organized, standardized process for data exchange across local, regional, and statewide healthcare IT initiatives

- Provides the means to reduce duplication of services with a resultant reduction of healthcare costs

- Facilitates reduced operational costs by enabling automation of many (currently manual) administrative tasks

- Provides governance and management over the data exchange process

The above benefits of an HIE demonstrate that collaboration and some type of alignment (as informal as it may be) between the participating providers are a subset of a successful exchange of patient information. Thus, while ARRA has not had an overall positive effect on the U.S. economy, it continues to promote healthcare IT application, clearly a needed feature toward achieving the long-term goals of accountable care.

Patient Protection and Affordable Care Act

On March 23, 2010, President Obama signed into law the Patient Protection and Affordable Care Act (PPACA) with the primary intention to provide insurance to all eligible U.S. citizens and to reduce personal healthcare expenditures. PPACA not only affects patients; it affects the medical community in many ways. This law is perhaps one of the most controversial statutes that has been politically fueled in many years. Numerous politicians and healthcare providers are unhappy with this law or with many of its provisions. Others are pleased with the increase in eligibility and the coverage PPACA provides. The general public seems con-fused and uncertain of its ramifications. Much of it is misunderstood by both political parties and consumers. But rather than discuss the pros and cons of

PPACA, the focus here is to highlight the effects it has had on physician-hospital alignment. A number of unanswered questions remain relative to the application of this law. Much more interpretation and clarification of PPACA's requirements will be necessary over the next few years as its tenets are implemented. Moreover, most of its effects will not take place until 2014 and beyond. Many of the provisions increase coverage levels, eliminate out-of-pocket expenses for some preventive care, and provide other financial benefits to patients across all levels of income. Some of the provisions increase taxes to certain types of healthcare providers and employers. However, there are some provisions that encourage physicians and hospitals to join together to improve patient care. Thus, the essence of alignment responds to this law and its current and prospective requirements.

The CMS ACO programs discussed earlier in this chapter were created under the PPACA. As outlined in that section, ACO entities provide an excellent opportunity for all physicians, hospitals, and other healthcare providers to align for improved quality of care, patient-centeredness, and reduction of costs. Additionally, Section 3502 of the PPACA provides grants to establish community-based interdisciplinary professional healthcare teams to support the PCMH endeavor. Virtually all of these new models of integration—PCMH, CIN, QC, and ACO—are largely a result of PPACA.

Established under the PPACA was a national Medicare pilot program to develop and evaluate paying a bundled payment for acute inpatient hospital services, physician services, outpatient hospital services, and post-acute care services for an episode of patient care that begins three days prior to a hospitalization and spans 30 days following discharge. Since the single bundled payment will cross over many different providers, in inpatient and outpatient settings, the participating providers will need to work together in the delivery of care and the allocation of the payment. This will be yet another form of alignment that varies from the ACOs and other models. Moreover, virtually all of the full integration physician-hospital alignment models plus the integrated entity structures (i.e., PCMH, CIN, ACO) are preparing for the inevitable changing reimbursement paradigm, which will ultimately lead to a bundled payment structure.

Summary

Regardless of ideology or political perspective, many have held for years that our current healthcare payment and delivery system is broken; that it delivers an inconsistent level of quality care, and in many cases, questionable value. Overall, healthcare providers in the United States function with great care and high professional standards, yet incentives have not been properly aligned. The focus has been on fee-for-service reimbursement, which emphasizes volume and not quality (even though most providers still perform services and make decisions for the good of the patient that are not motivated by economic gain). But the economic pressures along with legal liability risks incent providers to order more tests and do more rather than less. In turn, doing more still increases reimbursement and some believe this precludes physicians from focusing on their patients. Many aspects of healthcare reform, including the establishment of accountable care entities and PCMHs, encourage physicians and hospitals to collaborate on quality patient care.

Provider alignment, the use of EHR technology, and the exchange of patient information will blaze new trails on the road to improve healthcare in America. The merits of the recent laws surrounding healthcare reform is a debatable topic, and many unanswered questions must be resolved in the coming years. However, physician-hospital alignment will continue to be relevant and at the forefront of reform initiatives.

REFERENCES

1. *http://www.cdc.gov/nchs/data/hus/hus11.pdf#106,* accessed 8/23/2012.

2. *http://www.ncqa.org/tabid/631/default.aspx*, accessed 2/8/2012.

3. Although the relaxation of the Stark Law in 2007 allowed hospitals under certain conditions to provide up to 85% of the funding for an EHR system to a non-employed physician, relatively few hospitals or physicians chose to participate in this offering. With the increased incentive dollars under the CMS EHR incentive, more hospitals and physicians are taking advantage of the funding and joining together for the technology endeavor. The Stark relaxation provision expires 12/31/2013.

4. *http://www.himss.org/content/files/RHIO/RHIO_HIE_GeneralPresentation.pdf*, accessed 8/25/2012.

Alignment Models

Oftentimes, the words alignment and integration are used interchangeably when discussing working relationships between hospitals and physicians. Although they both fall into the same conceptual arena, the two terms are not one and the same. Alignment occurs when a physician or a private practice develops a professional relationship with a hospital or health system. Integration, however, is the approach taken for creating and implementing alignment strategies. There are three distinct levels of integration that should be considered, which are:

- Limited

- Moderate

- Full

As physicians and hospitals become clinically, financially, and technologically linked through alignment, the level of integration ultimately determines the scope of the relationship, the physicians' compensation for providing services, and the hospitals' financial outlay for receipt of these services.

A limited integration strategy describes a relationship that is relatively low in commitment and involvement wherein the parties are loosely tied together. To use the world of dating as an analogy for the different levels of integration, a limited integration model would be akin to two individuals who are "casually dating." Moving up one level along the continuum, a moderate integration structure represents a relationship that isn't fully financially tethered; however, it does provide additional forms of revenue for physicians and additional benefit to a health system. Again, in the dating game, this would entail a couple that is seriously dating but not yet ready to discuss marriage. Finally, a full integration model describes the highest form of integration in terms of commitment in which the physicians may or may not be employed by the hospital or health system; however, the relationship typically includes a significant amount (if not a majority) of the physicians' time being dedicated to performing services on behalf of their integration partner. If this were a couple, this integration level would represent the final step in the dating game: marriage. As detailed in the remainder of this chapter, within each level of integration, there are various structural models to consider.

Limited Integration Strategies

Managed care networks

Managed care networks include independent practice associations and physician hospital organizations. As we move into the accountable care era, these networks are being used as a platform for the development of accountable care organizations. However, these structures can also operate as a stand-alone alignment model. The basic concept behind the managed care network strategy is that it is comprised mainly of "loosely" formed alliances that are primarily for contracting purposes. Providers are able to gain some relief from economic burden by engaging in this strategy. However, these networks are generally limited in ability unless they become clinically integrated. By this we mean that they are normally no more than a messenger model with limited collaborative usefulness. Because of the nature of these agreements, the parties' loyalties are normally to the contract and not to each other. In this case, physician compensation could be affected if incentives received are distributed across the board. Otherwise, this level of integration generally does not have a true impact on compensation unless there are improvements in payer contracts.

Call coverage stipends

This particular strategy compensates physicians for the personal, financial, and risk burdens associated with their coverage of the emergency department. Physicians that participate in call coverage see all patients, both insured and noninsured, thereby causing them to request additional compensation from hospitals. Payment can come in the form of a daily stipend, fee-for-service, or through a hybrid payment method. As such, these can help alleviate some of the physicians' economic, personal, and liability burdens. The current trends for call coverage stipends show that other forms of alignment are becoming more pervasive, particularly for primary care physicians, who are generally not subject to a call coverage requirement as hospitalist programs now satisfy these needs.

Medical directorship

Basically, this model entails a physician being paid, usually at a market-based hourly rate, for carrying out defined administrative services at a healthcare organization under the requirement that there is a true need for these particular services. It is a separate contract from employment compensation contracts; and, because physicians are compensated on an hourly or per-service basis, it is necessary that they document hours worked and services provided. This is to avoid complications down the road, including any compliance issues that may arise from payment to physicians by hospitals for work that cannot be substantiated or is not documented. The main advantage of this model is that it is highly flexible to the needs of the organization: the organization can hire as many physicians as necessary to act as medical directors. Conversely, this model can potentially create political conflicts between the parties involved, and it does require a time commitment from the physicians. It is, however, a common alternative payment arrangement for a physician's administrative duties associated with his or her particular specialty/department.

Recruitment/incubation

A final example of a limited integration alignment strategy is recruitment/incubation. This refers to the traditional arrangement of a hospital financially supporting a new recruit. Hospitals may do this by providing income guarantees, offering tuition payments, creating an incubation model, or provider planning. The need for recruitment assistance must be substantiated by a community's need for such providers, and there are definitive regulations that hospitals must adhere to in providing these various recruitment support mechanisms. The compensation framework for this strategy allows existing physicians in practice to not experience a decrease in their pay as a new physician comes on board (and takes time to acclimate). Although this strategy offers flexibility once a need for it has been demonstrated by the healthcare organization, it may be short-lived as there are no guarantees of loyalty or collaboration from those newly recruited providers.

Moderate Integration Strategies

Management services organization

A management services organization (MSO) is created and owned by hospitals, private practices, private investors, or joint ventures to provide a myriad of services to its client practices. These services, which are mainly managerial or administrative in nature, can include revenue cycle, human resources, information technology, compliance, etc. This form of integration can provide an additional revenue stream for physicians and hospitals because it ties the hospitals to the physicians' business successes. Therefore, it has historically been an effective strategy to align with providers who are in private practice. However, it is worth noting that as the prevalence of private practice physicians decreases, the prevalence of MSO structures as a vehicle for alignment has also decreased. Regardless, it is important to note that the creation of an MSO must be done well, for not only is it a costly venture, it can also hurt the parties involved unless executed properly. As such, there are two aspects of consideration when forming a management services agreement between a qualified user and a service provider: the business side and the legal side.

On the business side, physicians and a hospital may potentially form a new entity ("NewCo") to provide specific management and administrative services. Typically structured as a limited liability company (LLC), NewCo hires or leases personnel necessary to provide management services. The purchaser of these services (either the hospital or physician office) pays NewCo a fair market management fee for providing these specified management services. This fee may be a fixed amount per month or a fixed percentage of revenues from services rendered; the actual payment structure is typically dependent on the scope of NewCo's responsibilities. The total compensation provided may also include performance incentives.

To remain viable on the legal side, NewCo must have a demonstrable benefit (cost or quality) as compared to the alternatives of the practice not pursuing the MSO strategy (i.e., going at in alone or involving a second party and developing a PHO). Also, with the percentage management fees, potential anti-kickback remains an issue as all fees paid must be commercially reasonable.

Equity model group assimilation

In this scenario, all entities in the alignment structure (typically a group of private practices) become tied together through legal arrangements. This allows all applicable parties to achieve high levels of efficiency and cost containment as they effectuate joint contracts with payers, which can yield increased profits for the physicians as a result of better contracts. Along the same lines, the parties are able to jointly develop ancillaries as well as marketing strategies.

Engaging in this model aligns the interests of all parties in relation to profitability and return on investment. Furthermore, it is easier and more efficient to administer one provider number as opposed to multiple. Nonetheless, this model does have some potential challenges that should be considered, particularly with respect to the transition phase. Some of these challenges include discussing and agreeing upon the governance structure, voting rights and procedures, and compensation for providers. Joint investments will be required, and return on those investments must be dependent upon the individual entity for there is no hospital subsidy. Overall, this model requires a high level of trust between all parties involved to be successful.

Provider equity

With a strategy that encompasses both joint ventures and provider investments, this option is for the more entrepreneurial physicians. Its main benefit is achieving a close union of parties under a common enterprise. For example, when physicians and hospitals effectuate a joint venture using this strategy, it usually leads to the development of specialized healthcare entities, such as specialty hospitals or surgery centers. Joint ventures are legally permissible if one of the following conditions is met:

- The physicians contribute financial capital

- The physicians provide business expertise

- The physicians have a business risk

Other structures of joint ventures include management services arrangements, real estate developments, freestanding centers, and even medical directorships. Needless to say, this strategy offers healthcare members a catalog of options for garnering additional economic benefits. Nonetheless, implementing such a strategy has proven to be challenging as it may be tricky to govern and increase operating costs once effectuated. However, when executed properly, this strategy can provide an additional stream of revenue to private practice physicians.

Target cost objectives and clinical co-management/ service line management

We conclude our discussion of moderate integration alignment models with an overview of two final strategies: target cost objectives and clinical co-management/ service line management. Target cost objectives is a program that focuses on ensuring the delivery of cost-effective care while still maintaining quality and patient satisfaction, two factors that are quickly gaining momentum in the current healthcare climate. Providers under this model receive a share of the savings realized by the hospital or health system as a result of their efforts. Compensation can either be a percentage of the savings, an hourly rate, or a fixed fee. Physicians are integral in the planning process for this model to determine how these savings can be actualized; otherwise, all parties involved face potentially detrimental challenges. Furthermore, this model is not meant as a long-term alignment solution.

The clinical co-management/service line management strategy is another popular and highly recommended option in the healthcare industry. The purpose of clinical co-management/service line management arrangements is to reward physicians for their efforts in developing, managing, and improving the quality and efficiency of a particular hospital service line. It is a contractual relationship between the hospital and the physician management entity—often a physician practice, or potentially even a group of physicians from different practices—that engages physicians in the provision of administrative services and works toward certain strategic initiatives within that service line. For example, orthopedic surgery is a specialty that commonly utilizes clinical co-management arrangements, as there are often savings that can be realized relative to implants and other devices. Participants of this model—both hospitals and physicians—can realize strong economic returns and strategic alignment opportunities. Also, if necessary, this alignment model can be easier to unwind through a termination of the existing contractual agreement. This model can be utilized in several different arrangements and contracts, including:

- **Management agreements:** This is a typical structure for an arrangement between a health system and a single, existent physician practice. (Model A)

- **Newly created management entities:** Typically utilized when several practices will be part of the clinical co-management efforts; often, a new entity is created that includes all participating physicians, rather than the hospital executing agreements with each participating practice. (Model B)

- **Joint venture management entities:** Sometimes, the hospital and physician practice will develop a joint venture that will oversee and manage all parties' involvement in this process. (Model C)

- **Joint oversight committee:** This structure includes development of a dedicated governance committee to oversee multiple practices' participation in the clinical co-management agreement. Individual management agreements are typically executed between the hospital and participating practices within this structure. (Model D)

For further description of these four potential structural models, see Figure 4.1.

Effectuating an alignment strategy through a contractual relationship (as opposed to an employment arrangement) can be complex as it requires strong combined vision and agreement on strategic goals and operating principles. Despite the type of contract or arrangement, all four possible forms of clinical co-management

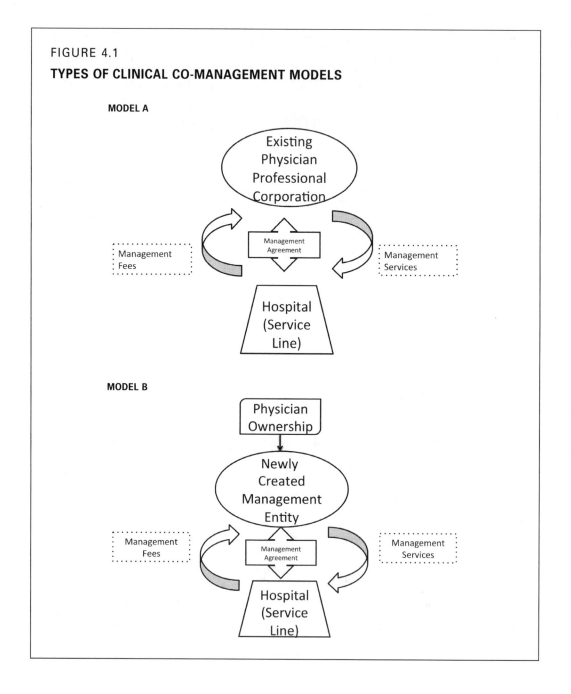

FIGURE 4.1

TYPES OF CLINICAL CO-MANAGEMENT MODELS

MODEL A

Existing Physician Professional Corporation

Management Fees

Management Agreement

Management Services

Hospital (Service Line)

MODEL B

Physician Ownership

Newly Created Management Entity

Management Fees

Management Agreement

Management Services

Hospital (Service Line)

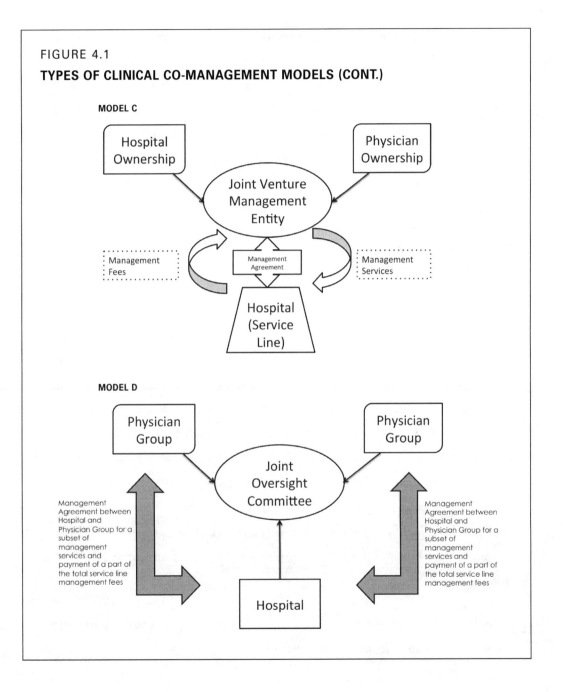

FIGURE 4.1

TYPES OF CLINICAL CO-MANAGEMENT MODELS (CONT.)

MODEL C

Hospital Ownership

Physician Ownership

Joint Venture Management Entity

Management Fees

Management Agreement

Management Services

Hospital (Service Line)

MODEL D

Physician Group

Physician Group

Joint Oversight Committee

Management Agreement between Hospital and Physician Group for a subset of management services and payment of a part of the total service line management fees

Management Agreement between Hospital and Physician Group for a subset of management services and payment of a part of the total service line management fees

Hospital

The Healthcare Executive's Guide to Physician-Hospital Alignment

agreements entail a provider or a group of providers rendering services (e.g., clinical, management, and other services) for a specific inpatient or outpatient service line with a hospital, in turn, providing them with remuneration in line with fair market value (FMV) and commercially reasonable standards. These payments typically include an hourly rate (at FMV) for administrative time and incentive payments for achieving established service line metrics. Incentive payments may be performance-based in part and/or tied to achievement of specific quality objectives.

Full Integration Strategies

Employment

Traditionally, a common form of full integration (and also the tightest alignment strategy) has been employment wherein physicians become employees of a hospital or integrated health system. An IRS W-2 employment agreement solidifies this relationship and outlines the terms by which the physicians will function and be compensated. In this capacity, physicians have full benefits provided by the hospital, they must abide by standard employee regulations, and taxes and social security are withheld. The compensation framework for hospital-employed providers typically is a productivity payment with potential financial incentives for achieving quality or cost control. At the outset of employment, it is also common for a hospital to provide guaranteed compensation. Typically this lasts for no longer than three years.

The structure for employment may vary based on the needs and capacities of the hospital. For example, larger hospitals may establish two channels of employment:

one for their primary care network and another for their specialty care providers. Some hospitals may create a new department and employ all physicians within that specific department; others may set up a separate legal entity or subsidiary, or even a foundation to employ physicians.

Although employment by a hospital or health system increases the potential for job security and minimizes the physicians' economic risk, physicians have far less flexibility under this model than with others.

Professional services agreement

Often referred to as "employment lite," the professional services agreement (PSA) model has come to the forefront as consolidation becomes increasingly more prevalent within the healthcare industry. In comparison to an employment strategy, the PSA model allows the practice to remain private while hedging payer risk. This model falls just short of full employment but still represents a high level of physician-hospital integration. Physicians participating in this model are contracted to the hospital on an IRS 1099 Form status, and this relationship is formalized by a PSA. In this case, the hospital contracts with these physicians for various services, which may be either clinical (professional) services or non-clinical (administrative) services. Often, additional components such as call coverage and payment for quality outcomes are included in the overall PSA structure. Under the PSA, the hospital owns all receivables but will provide the physicians with payment that covers physician compensation and benefits and other overhead costs incurred. As such, the hospital may choose to compensate physicians on a productivity basis, often by using physician work relative value units (wRVU). Payment for additional components may take other forms (such as a daily stipend or variable amount, based on outcomes), per the terms of the agreement.

There are four basic variations on the PSA model that are the most recognized and commonly used. These four scenarios are as follows:

- Global payment PSA: The hospital contracts with the practice for services in exchange for a global payment rate, which includes all physician compensation and any potential bonuses as well as all practice overhead expenses. Further, the practice retains all management responsibilities and continues to employ its staff. The practice functions as an independent contractor, thereby receiving no benefits from the hospital. The practice invoices the hospital for all contracted services rendered (and for any professional fees associated with other services performed at and for the hospital) and files a Form 1099 with the IRS signifying practice responsibility for withholding taxes from its physicians. Ancillaries may be leased or sold to the hospital at FMV rates.

- Practice management arrangement: The hospital employs physicians; the practice entity is retained and contracts with the hospital for management services. Administrative management staff members are not employed by the hospital, as the practice provides these services via a management contract (another agreement) and receives a corresponding fee.

- Traditional PSA: The hospital contracts with physicians (their historical practice entity) for professional services; the hospital employs staff and "owns" administrative structure. Ancillaries are usually acquired by the hospital within this model.

- Hybrid arrangements: The hospital both employs and contracts with physicians. The practice entity spins off into a jointly owned MSO/information services organization; various scenarios involving mixing and matching of services (both professional and administrative) exist.

The PSA arrangement can offer physicians and hospitals a plethora of options and flexibility for meeting the needs of all those involved. Above all, physicians are able to retain their independence while gaining the opportunity to increase their bottom line and forge a stable relationship with a hospital. This model also provides the opportunity for an easy segue to full employment should it ever be desired or necessary.

Summary

Alignment has afforded providers and hospitals the ability to respond to the shifting healthcare climate as well as their ever-changing needs. Historically, many physicians have perceived alignment to be synonymous with employment. As this chapter has demonstrated, employment is not the only option for alignment—nor should it be.

It is important to remember that every model carries with it advantages and disadvantages. To maximize the benefits of the alignment model, it is imperative to first decide which strategy is the best fit for your organization and how to best implement it. There are also legal aspects and ramifications associated with every model that must be considered during and after implementation, which are discussed in more detail in Chapter 9. Nonetheless, the diverse array of alignment models within each level of integration can offer both providers and hospitals viable solutions to many of the challenges they are facing in healthcare today.

Alignment Strategies

Prior chapters in this book have discussed what physician alignment is, defined the models, and presented some of the challenges associated with alignment for both physicians and hospitals. This chapter dives deeper into the specific alignment models that are commonly used and when they are most applicable as strategies. Over the past two to three years, as the alignment trend has continued to grow throughout the healthcare provider industry, the specific characteristics of the different models have evolved, as various tweaks and refinements are made to better fit each individual scenario. In the typical market, a number of alignment strategies have emerged as predominant solutions that many physician groups and health systems have embraced. Still, new approaches are being developed in regard to how hospitals and physicians approach alignment, so it is clear that we have just begun to see what will ultimately unfold relative to integration.

Continuum of Alignment Strategies

While a variety of alignment models are available for both hospitals and physicians to explore and pursue, all fall somewhere on a continuum, with the lesser-aligned models on the far left and full alignment versions on the opposite end of the spectrum. (See Figure 5.1 for the continuum of alignment strategies.) Each individual alignment strategy includes its own degree of risk, investment, and difficulty that stakeholders involved must consider; however, the majority of the specific models fall somewhere in between these two extremes. And despite the fact that the larger deals and those that are often in the spotlight relate more to employment and similar transaction models, there are many alignment transactions between hospitals and physicians about which most people never hear of or even realize that an affiliation has occurred.

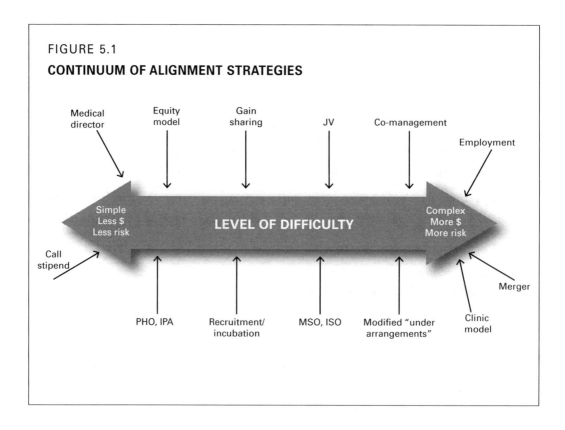

FIGURE 5.1

CONTINUUM OF ALIGNMENT STRATEGIES

The Healthcare Executive's Guide to Physician-Hospital Alignment

Indeed, some of the best alignment models achieved between hospitals and physicians over the past few years are those that have remained completely unknown to the public. Primarily, the first wave of physician-hospital consolidation in the 1990s and early 2000s was founded on one model, and this involved a relatively large transaction providing up-front payouts to the seller to bring its practice under a hospital's network and brand.

The current wave of consolidation, referred to as alignment or physician-hospital partnerships, offers many models that both sides of the deal can pursue to achieve their desired outcome, without major imbalances and with win-win solutions for both parties. Today's trends of physician alignment is not a zero sum game, in terms of winners and losers, and if the deals are done right with both parties coming to the table as partners, it is most likely that both sides will emerge as winners from their alignment strategy. Being partners, however, is a very different tone from what many physicians and hospitals have had in past alignment discussions. To further complicate matters, both sides are still carrying with them baggage from some poorly executed deal that took place 15 years ago or more.

In today's alignment trends, some of the most successfully executed deals are those that provide healthy degrees of ongoing independence among the parties involved in the partnership. This often means allowing the practice to keep its name and deliver services the same way it did when it was independent. It may also mean continuing to allow the practice to conduct its own revenue cycle management (i.e., billing and collections) because hospitals that will likely be most effective in operating ambulatory operations are those that admit they are not structured to do ambulatory billing. And in some cases, this may mean keeping the practice fully independent, with the hospital contracting through a formal arrangement. (We will discuss this later in the chapter relative to professional services agreements.) Regardless of the model the parties choose and the valuation placed on this transaction, unless both sides come together as partners, the likelihood of the venture's success will become a challenge very quickly.

Employment as an Alignment Strategy

The most well-known and perhaps commonly seen alignment strategy in the market today is employment. Within the past three to five years, hospitals have rapidly returned to the prospect of employing physicians as a primary model for alignment. Although many hospitals keenly recall their past experiences with employing physicians and how most of them proved unsuccessful/unsustainable to varying degrees, the current cycle of physician employment by hospitals has already proven to be different.

Most employment situations have two distinct components to the overall transaction. First, there is the actual employment of each individual physician in a particular group, which is solidified via an employment agreement. Second, there is the acquisition of the physician's medical practice, which is effectuated through an asset purchase agreement.

Practice acquisition is relatively straightforward. Due to the various regulations and requirements relating to fair market value (FMV) payments between hospitals and physicians, as well as the fact that the majority of medical practices have very little, if any, intangible value in their businesses, the hospitals typically purchase only the practice's tangible assets in an employment transaction. This means that the hospital will most likely not pay the practice's shareholders (i.e., physician partners) any goodwill or intangible value for their practice, even though physicians will argue that such value does exist in their business.

An acquisition of the practice's tangible assets typically includes furniture, fixtures, and equipment of any sort within the practice, owned by the practice. Leased equipment or supplies are excluded from the assets; and, in most cases, any real estate owned by the practice's partner(s) is separated as well. Usually where a practice's physicians own their real estate, the actual property is typically owned through a separate entity, such as a limited liability company (LLC) or other type of limited liability partnership. As a part of the transaction, it is possible that the hospital is interested in purchasing the real estate; however, there are different variables to consider in a real estate transaction, compared to the employment and practice acquisition. With real estate transactions, there are different comparables used in appraisals, as well as entirely different valuation approaches. These are typically conducted by specific real estate appraisers, and the valuations will have less of a specific application or consideration of the nature of the business and thus will be based more on the factors impacting the local commercial real estate market. Also, depending on the nature of the transaction being considered, it may be necessary to determine a FMV lease rate for the property in question, which in and of itself includes multiple specific components, such as monthly rental rates per square foot, tenant improvements, local taxes, market lease rate comparables, etc. As such, the real estate will typically be completed through a separate transaction, which appraises the property appropriately and is effectuated with the actual LLC or entity that owns the property.

Overall, the process for valuing the practice's tangible assets in the employment/
asset purchase transaction is relatively straightforward. A formal FMV opinion is
completed, typically by a third-party appraiser, such as a consulting or financial
services firm that is experienced in healthcare entity transactions. This opinion
involves the valuator conducting an inventory of the tangible assets, and providing an opinion on FMV that the hospital should pay the practice for each
individual asset being purchased.

In some employment transactions, hospitals will include a certain degree of
goodwill to be paid to the physician partners in the practice. This can sometimes
be affected through workforce-in-place, which essentially compensates the sellers
for the intrinsic value associated with the practice's people and costs associated
with building their business, all of which are critical in the practice's market
value. Some hospitals will also pay for medical records, which are always based
on a rate per record and should solely include active patient charts. Although
some other methods of paying for goodwill have been observed, these payments
can be challenging to fall into compliance with FMV and commercially reasonableness standards; as such, they are typically avoided in employment scenarios.

While the asset purchase component of employment transactions are, for the most
part, relatively straightforward, the actual employment contract is typically a little
more complicated. *Note:* We typically refer to the process of a hospital employing
a physician as a transaction, even though people do not view their employment as
a transaction, such as a transaction to buy or sell a vehicle. However, in the case of
a hospital employing a physician, the parts that make up the deal comprise a
transaction to buy a physician's business.

Indeed, in an employment alignment, the physician partners truly are selling their business. The majority of transactions involving the sale of a private company to a larger organization typically comprise two components:

- The up-front payment for the business enterprise.

- The earn-out, which obligates the management to stay in the business for a certain period of time and achieve defined performance levels before they can get a certain amount of the overall transaction value. The employment component of the physician alignment transaction is akin to an earn-out.

In most employment models, the physician is agreeing to being employed exclusively by the hospital for a time frame of typically three to five years. Further, his or her compensation is typically based on certain defined levels of performance, as is addressed in further detail below. One thing that is unique about physician employment as compared to other private businesses is that the amount of the transaction paid up front is most often relatively minor since, as we previously discussed, the hospital is only purchasing the tangible assets. Even if the hospital does pay for goodwill, it still will not represent the bulk of the true value of the physicians' services that comprised that medical practice business. Therefore, the bulk of the value paid to the physicians in an employment scenario is paid through the physician's ongoing compensation that he or she is projected to receive under his or her employment with the hospital. This is the physician's earn-out of sorts, even though we typically refer to it as an employment contract.

Another unique aspect of employment arrangements is that the overall model that makes up the various components of the physician's compensation can be quite complex. In order for the hospital to provide a comparable level of compensation growth and comply with FMV limitations, the hospital has to find multiple pathways—albeit legitimate and entirely legal—to compensate the physician for his or her services.

The most basic element of physician compensation under employment arrangements is typically based on a guaranteed base salary, with a productivity-based bonus model. For primary care physicians, this is often straightforward, because their most common reason for pursuing employment with a hospital is to prevent their income levels from declining (as they most likely have seen in private practice settings in recent years) and then perhaps receive some level of income growth throughout their employment period. When a physician practice sells to a hospital and the partners become employed, this is rarely a situation of the physician selling out the business and retiring to the beach.

Hospitals can often provide income security, reduction in risks, and possibly moderate income growth, based on corresponding productivity/performance growth. However, they can rarely, if ever, provide liquidity to shareholders without any corresponding performance on the back end through employment over an extended period of time. Without the physician performing at historical productivity levels, there is little value to the hospital for entering into that arrangement, and from a compliance standpoint, it will most likely raise red flags.

Employment compensation models will often incorporate a reasonable base salary for the physician, which the hospital can guarantee for the first two years of the employment, and possibly extend through the third year as well. It is not reasonable for a hospital to guarantee a physician's salary for all five years of a contract, due to the fact that beyond the third year, there are too many variables that could impact the model, which would, in turn, require adjustments or an altogether new structure for the contract. In many cases, the base will be less than the physician's prior year's salary; though, this is not to say that he or she should expect to receive less compensation under employment.

Beyond the base salary, there is typically a bonus incentive, which is most often based on the physician's productivity. The physician's productivity is often measured by his or her physician work relative value units (wRVU), which is a method of tracking the physician's individually performed professional services, while controlling for other variables that will change from physician to physician. This allows different physicians to be compared on an apples-to-apples basis, which does not fluctuate depending on the patients' insurance, the practice's payer mix and managed care contracts, market/patient demographics, or how well the practice bills and collects for its services.

Measuring wRVUs is the purest form of measuring what a physician does and the amount he or she performs those services, compared to applicable benchmarks representing the physician's cohort and geographic marketplace. And since wRVUs are set and adjusted annually by the Centers for Medicare & Medicaid Services (CMS), the true value of the physician's services is reflected in the fee schedule that is used as the standard for comparison throughout the nation each year.

The bonus incentive component of the compensation often allows the physician to achieve his or her historical level of compensation with reasonable increases in the prior year's income. However, it is a bonus because it requires that the physician fulfills a defined level of performance, which in most cases will be consistent with the physician's historical level of wRVU productivity. Moreover, if the physician increases his or her productivity levels, which is often possible after being employed by a hospital, he or she can achieve even larger compensation increases, since the fixed costs of employment have been covered and the physician's productivity justifies such increases.

This model is often appealing to many internal medicine/primary care physicians, as well as numerous specialty physicians that have experienced financial challenges resulting from reimbursement cuts in the past because it provides income stability with the hospital, while providing incentive opportunity for the physician. That bonus income is based on a simple structure, whereby once the physician's base overhead and fixed costs are covered, the physician can achieve more compensation per wRVU for incremental amounts of wRVUs beyond a base threshold. This compensation per wRVU ratio is referred to as the *conversion factor* and it essentially provides more bang for the physician's buck on every wRVU beyond the base.

A variety of employment compensation models are in use; this is a common approach because it provides the income stability for the physician, along with opportunities for greater income if his or her productivity justifies it. Such approaches are growing in popularity with physicians, due to the fact that once the physician is employed and his or her income is based solely on wRVU productivity, he or she no longer has to be concerned about running a medical practice, billing and collections, or patients' insurance. This becomes the responsibility of the hospital and any deficiencies in the hospital's ability to run the business and financial side of a practice will not impact the physician's take-home income.

The physicians can focus on what they were trained to do: see patients and focus on providing the highest quality of care with undivided attention.

Professional Services Agreements as an Alignment Strategy

After employment, perhaps the most common physician-hospital alignment model occurring in today's healthcare marketplace is the professional services agreement (PSA). While the term is not new within the business of healthcare delivery, the PSA model used as a form of alignment between hospitals and physicians currently taking place is new and significantly different. As presented in Chapter 4, we often refer to PSAs as "employment lite" arrangements, in that they are similar to employment in terms of the mechanics of the deal; however, these models allow for continued independence and separation for the physicians from the hospital, thus making them easier to unwind if necessary. And while it has taken a couple of years for the PSA model to really gain traction, it is now extremely popular with many physician group practices and hospitals are embracing it as a method for investing in effective, long-term arrangements with practices representing significant strategic value.

From 2009 to 2011, the PSA was commonly seen in hospital arrangements with cardiologists and practices specializing in cardiac services. The reason for this was because cardiac ancillary services received significant reimbursement cuts during this time, which made the cardiology medical practice model unsustainable. Among other challenges these cuts created for cardiologists, the largest was the fact that many of them could no longer operate their office-based ancillary and diagnostic services for profit. As such, pursuing alignment with a hospital was the sole alternative for many cardiology providers throughout the country. And while many of them did end up taking the employment route, the PSA turned out to be a much more attractive model for a large number of cardiology practices that wanted to eliminate risks associated with their ancillaries while at the same time achieving greater stability in their income.

In the current market phase, however, we have moved beyond cardiology PSA deals, partially because the majority of cardiologists have now pursued some sort of alignment model with hospitals. But, as the PSA model has become more accepted by hospitals, these deals are now taking place with other providers, including a wide range of specialties and even primary care in some instances. As a result of this growth, the PSA is rapidly becoming one of the most popular alignment models within the market today.

Just like with employment, there are a number of specific ways that a PSA can be structured. Most often, these deals are structured in two key parts:

- The hospital purchases 100% of a group's practice-based ancillaries (i.e., their technical component services)

- The hospital contracts with the practice through the PSA for all professional services

Since various surgical specialty groups have started to pursue PSA arrangements with hospitals in greater numbers, a third element has emerged, which relates to when there is a separate ambulatory surgery center (ASC) owned by the practice's physicians. When this is the case, the hospital will usually purchase a stake in the

ASC at FMV, where the specific amount of equity purchased by the hospital will vary depending on that state's regulatory requirements for such transactions.

Most PSA deals involve a three-year agreement, wherein the hospital compensates a group of physicians for all professional services performed within the practice. All ownership of the practice remains with the physicians, except for the ancillaries purchased by the hospital. This can sometimes be tricky, depending on the types of ancillaries that a practice has; however, if these services can be effectively segmented out of the practice, then it makes sense for the hospital to purchase those ancillaries at FMV. The value for the hospital owning these ancillaries will come when they can bill under hospital outpatient department rates, which will be higher than when billing those same services under the practice.

Separate from the purchase of the practice's ancillaries is the PSA payment from the hospital to the physicians, and the most popular method of structuring this payment is through the PSA global fee model. This payment is based on a global fee, which is determined by a global rate, or the physicians' fee per wRVU. The calculation of the global fee is multiplying the total number of the physicians' wRVUs for a defined period (i.e., quarterly) by the global rate, which is a FMV figure compared to national benchmarks.

The global fee is designed to cover both the practice's professional-related overhead (i.e., excluding ancillary-related expenses, which are now owned by the hospital) and the physicians' compensation. The payment for the practice's professional overhead is most often based on a simple pass-through of those expenses incurred to the hospital. In some cases, the payment designated for the practice's expenses related to professional services is based on a budget that would be established by the practice and agreed upon by the hospital. When the PSA follows this approach, the practice is responsible for ensuring its costs remain within that budgeted amount; if the costs are greater, then those overages come out of the physician fee portion. Conversely, if there is a margin of profit between the portion of the global fee covering professional overhead and the actual costs of that overhead, then those funds are distributed to the physicians (or otherwise invested in the practice). It is important that the global fee and budgeted overhead portion are reasonable such that any profits that do result for the practice will not jeopardize the deal's compliance with FMV standards.

The remainder of the global fee after professional overhead is covered goes to the physicians' compensation, just as it does in a private practice model, where compensation is derived from the practice's profit from operations. However, under the PSA with the hospital, physicians' income is now based on their levels of wRVU productivity, rather than being dictated by the multiple variables that often drag down their actual compensation in the private practice setting, such as poorly managed care contracts, reimbursement cuts, inefficient billing, and collections.

The physician fee portion of the PSA's global fee can often entail a compensation increase for the physicians each year of the PSA from their prior years' compensation in private practice. The amount ultimately going to the physicians in the PSA deal must still comply with all FMV and commercially reasonableness guidelines. As such, any compensation increases for the physicians under the PSA compared to their historical income must be reasonable and all of their compensation under the PSA should be linked to the physicians' individual productivity levels.

That being the case, however, the global fee is typically paid as a lump sum to the physicians and the global rate is based on a total number of wRVUs among all the physicians in the practice. So, once the PSA payment is made by the hospital to the practice, the practice's physician partners then have full discretion as to how those funds are distributed to individual members. This means that the physician compensation portion of the global fee can be allocated equally among the physicians, or the partners can establish and follow another income distribution model that incorporates other variables, such as physicians' individual productivity contribution to the wRVU pool. If such a distribution model is developed, certain physicians will receive more compensation compared to others within the same group; however, the hospital will most likely not have involvement in setting those actual distribution structures (because the physicians have full discretion in distributing those funds).

In addition to the core components of most PSA deals previously described in the global fee PSA model, there are typically a number of other aspects of the overall PSA alignment transaction that dictate how the relationship should function for the hospital and the physician. For instance, there is typically a management committee established, which is composed of equal representation from the practice and hospital, and this committee fulfills the general governance and performance oversight of the arrangement on a regular basis. Figure 5.2 highlights common PSA structures.

Aside from the management committee, another common component of PSA deals is a management agreement for billing of the ancillary services. Since most hospitals are not well versed in ambulatory or provider-based billing and since the practice is already set up for the billing of both professional and ancillary services,

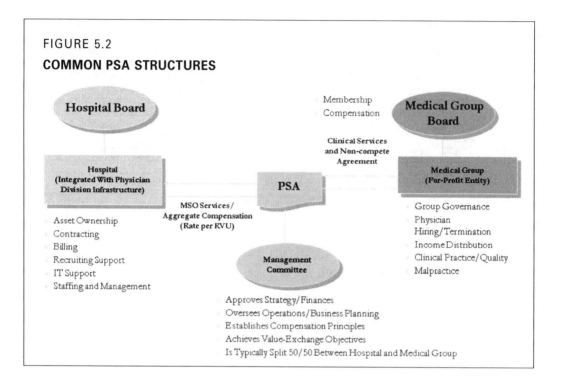

FIGURE 5.2

COMMON PSA STRUCTURES

it often makes sense for that function to remain within the practice. As such, the hospital can pay the practice a FMV fee for continuing to manage the billing and collections of the practice-based ancillaries, which are being acquired by the hospital in the deal. This fee is often based on a percentage of collections, just as an outside billing company would typically structure such fees, and this fee would be separate from the other components of the overall PSA transaction.

Although the basic conceptual components of PSAs are quite simple and relatively direct, some of the PSA deals occurring in the marketplace today can often be complex. In this regard, many PSA deals, particularly those involving larger specialty and multi-specialty groups, have become more like the multifaceted structured deals often seen in larger company mergers. Moreover, the overall valuations associated with many of these transactions have also grown to be quite significant, where a PSA deal between a hospital and large specialty practice with significant ancillaries can exceed $50 million in total transaction value.

The more complex aspects of these deals typically come in when the ancillaries being purchased by the hospital are heavily integrated with the professional component of the practice (as most practices are structured), thus requiring those components to be extracted from the practice going forward. It can also become more complex when structuring PSA arrangements with multi-specialty group practices because this will create the need for different rates per wRVU within each individual specialty.

Despite the various complexities that sometimes emerge within PSA transactions, this model has proven to generate a great deal of advantages for both the practice's physicians and the hospital. Initially, PSAs were considered more of an interim option for cardiologists who needed a one-to-three-year solution that would provide some stability until something could be done to prevent the government's recommended reimbursement cuts from becoming permanent. The idea was that a PSA would be much easier to reverse or unravel when and if the physicians wanted to separate from the hospital in the future, compared to unraveling an employment arrangement, which is extremely difficult to do without significant investments and outside resources.

However, PSA deals have gone on to reflect significant benefits for both sides, and the majority of these initial transactions are being extended or renewed as they approach the end of their initial three-year terms. The prior success of these arrangements has also spawned an entire wave of new alignment transactions, which often involve physician groups that were not really pursuing hospital alignment before.

Other Alignment Strategies

Aside from the employment and PSA models, hospitals and physicians are pursuing a number of other specific strategies as methods of aligning more closely. Keep in mind, we typically view alignment on a continuum, with full alignment on the far right end comprising employment and PSAs. In the middle are moderate forms of alignment, ultimately continuing all the way to the left of the continuum where lesser forms of alignment are classified. And while employment and PSAs comprise a large portion of the focus behind alignment and involve actual transactions between the hospital and physicians, the lesser and moderate forms of alignment have been pervasive throughout the healthcare market for several years, even before full alignment came into the spotlight.

Two moderate forms of alignment that have become more popular in the past couple of years are service line management and clinical co-management agreements. Also, various joint venture (JV) arrangements have continued to become more common, such as those that involve the hospital purchasing an equity stake in a practice's ASC. In these instances, the hospital essentially becomes a silent capital partner with the physicians in the ASC venture, as opposed to playing a more active role in the facility's operations. However, these JVs still create a formalized affiliation between the hospital and the physician, which provides value for the physicians through the hospital's capital investment, and value for the hospital is derived through the closer relationship with the physicians.

Service line management arrangements entail less involved, albeit still formalized agreements between a hospital and a group of physicians, whereby the physicians provide certain management functions for defined services within the hospital. The compensation to the physicians for delivering these services is typically paid via a stipend (hourly or daily) and is shared as a total pool among the full group of doctors participating in the agreement. The value for both sides of these arrangements typically lies in the ability of the physicians to inject certain financial benefits for the hospital, which the hospital is permitted to share alongside the physicians. As such, the compensation to the physicians under service line management agreements is "at risk," in that the hospital only pays the physicians a portion of the financial gains achieved through the initiatives defined under the physicians' responsibilities.

Somewhat similar to service line management arrangements are clinical co-management agreements. And while the general concept behind service line management arrangements are quite commonly practiced, clinical co-management agreements are newer, more formalized models of alignment. Clinical co-management agreements are often established through the creation of a separate entity owned by the physicians, which is contracted to provide certain services to the hospital. These services are related to the management and oversight of a specific clinical department or division within a hospital's department, whereas service line management agreements are more related to administrative and operational management functions of a specific service line, which can be either within a primary department of the hospital or externally connected through the hospital's medical staff.

Another key difference between these two models is that the physicians' compensation under clinical co-management is typically not based on any sort of gain-sharing arrangement. In other words, the compensation is not based on increased value that may have come from any savings or otherwise improvements that came about from the physician's work under the agreement. Such "shared savings" can be used to justify a certain amount of compensation to the phyhsicians; however, these are typically separate groups entirely, and thus not implemented in clinical co-management agreements. The hospital can pay physicians for a number of tasks under clinical co-management agreements based on a set fee that is independently determined to be FMV and often will be based on an hourly or daily rate. However, any payments that are made to the physicians must be based on legitimately performed and tracked work completed by the participating physicians. This work will always be performed separately from and in addition to the physicians' standard professional, diagnostic, surgical, or otherwise technical encounters with patients.

And finally, in discussing various alignment strategies, we cannot ignore the limited forms of alignment, most of which are not new concepts and are often strategies that physicians and hospitals have been partnering on for a number of years. In today's competitive marketplace where the most critical component of a hospital's existence lies in the quality of its physician network, these limited alignment models are proving to be extremely valuable for both parties—the hospital and the physicians—in establishing partnerships that yield beneficial results without requiring major outlays or burdensome risk. These limited models are especially attractive for those hospitals that do not have the capital/operational resources to execute a larger transaction that is often required for PSAs or to invest the capital resources in building extensive employed physician resources that would be required to achieve reasonable critical mass.

Examples of limited alignment strategies include among others: medical directorships, pay-for-call arrangements, and teaching-related contracts within academic hospitals. We will not spend a great amount of time on these limited alignment model strategies here, since most of them are addressed in other chapters of this book. For now, the most critical aspect related to most of these arrangements is that the compensation allocated to participating physicians is market-based and most involve a FMV hourly rate. Thus, payments are distributed based on the hourly rate and an actual number of hours where work was specifically performed.

Pay-for-call arrangements are somewhat unique, however, in that these agreements involve the hospital compensating physicians simply providing call coverage, regardless of whether he or she was actually called to come into the hospital during that time. The concept of pay-for-call has sparked the most controversy of all the alignment strategies discussed in this text and typically has varying support from health system executives as to whether they should have to compensate members of their medical staff simply for providing call coverage. It is even more controversial for those hospitals that face the challenge of entering into pay-for-call arrangements with certain specialists, which in turn will motivate other members of the medical staff to seek out similar arrangements, ultimately resulting in the hospital having to possibly pay all of its physicians to provide call coverage or face losing that coverage as a consequence.

Despite the controversy surrounding pay-for-call as an alignment model, this is a reality for many hospitals that have difficulties covering emergency department call for a comprehensive range of specialties. As such, pay-for-call arrangements have become relatively common and have ultimately pushed the federal government to render specific guidelines surrounding how a hospital can compensate physicians for providing call coverage. And while these arrangements involve more unique parameters compared to some other alignment models, all pay-for-call agreements must comply with the applicable regulations related to FMV and commercial reasonableness guidelines.

Summary

As the concept of physician alignment becomes more mainstream, the specific characteristics of the many alignment transactions occurring within various markets throughout the country continue to evolve. This evolution in alignment models encompasses a wide variation in payments for services under various arrangements, as well as a general increase in the innovation and creativity behind how many of these transactions are being structured.

We are, perhaps, at the cusp of physician alignment emerging, and as more groups seek affiliations and the population of buyers/partners continues to expand, it is safe to assume that the nature of these transactions will continue to evolve as well. Employment will continue to be a strong theme throughout the alignment trend. In our modern environment of clinical integration and evolution toward accountable care, it will continue to make sense for hospitals to employ certain physicians.

Yet, as more hospital executives realize that employment is not the only route, they will continue to be flexible to alternative affiliation models. Moreover, perhaps the most compelling driver of this trend will be the physicians, in that more individual medical providers will understand that they do not have to sell their practice completely and become an employee of a single health system. Other alternative structures are available for aligning with these hospitals, each of which entails varying degrees of connectivity.

Physician Practice Perspective

What do physicians want and need from their practices, and what are their reasons for aligning with hospitals and health systems? We mentioned some of these needs briefly in Chapter 1, and will now discuss them in more detail.

Physician-hospital alignment calls for an understanding of what physicians want and need. The focus of this chapter is to differentiate the physicians' "wants" from their "needs" and to compare them with the hospitals' perspective, as will later be addressed in Chapter 7. Interestingly, their views are similar, just from different perspectives. The hospital needs competent physicians; a practice needs a competent hospital in order to continue providing quality patient care and services. The geographic community covered by the proposed alignment depends on the same competency from the hospital.

For an alignment to be effective in providing services, the hospital must present an organized competent nursing staff, allied health providers, and hospital administration support staff. Having an attractive and efficient physical plant and diagnostic equipment available is as important (if not more important) to the physicians as it is to the hospital. Lastly, as is addressed in Chapter 7, the hospital's desire for increased volumes and improvement in financial results are equally important to the physician.

Physicians' wants and needs include:

- Security and stability

- Respect and appreciation

- Adequate market share

- Continuing education and training

- Participation in managed care plans

- Financial support and compensation

- Access to capital

- Work-life balance

Security and Stability

As physicians review hospital alignment opportunities, they seek continued and enhanced financial and practice security. They strive for lasting stability and consistency. They consider the facilities that are available for adequate space to perform their services today and in the future. Ultimately, physicians desire practice security for the following reasons:

- To achieve and maintain fair compensation that is aligned with productivity

- To ensure their compensation is compliant with fair market value

- To be incentivized and rewarded for their continued efforts and hard work

Respect and Appreciation

All people want to feel needed, appreciated, and respected, and physicians are no different. Physicians would like to see critical communication tactics implemented to effect two-way communication. For true alignment, both hospitals and physicians will require a consistent ongoing dialogue. This dialogue will help build mutual trust between the hospital administration and the physicians.

A good way for hospitals and physicians to connect personally and professionally is to establish a set monthly meeting between the CEO and individual physicians. (Other members of the hospital's leadership team, such as the COO, CFO, chief nursing officer, and the specific individual responsible for the physician network, likely the director of the physician practices or physician network CEO, should also hold regular meetings with individual physicians.) This regular meeting is a good time to find out what is going on with physicians on a personal level. The CEO should ask about physicians' families or upcoming vacations.

When meeting with physicians, administration should show their concern and sincerity, demonstrating genuine respect. Ask the physicians, "What is going well?" or "Are there any personal issues that may affect your performance?" Administrators may be surprised what they hear from physicians. This is a good time for the physician to say that the nursing staff has been extremely helpful during a code, or possibly they might express appreciation for seeing the CEO rounding on the floors. Physicians like to brag about the hospital, but sometimes with their busy schedules, they may not have an appropriate venue for expressing what is going well.

Another simple, but valuable, question to ask is, "Do you have the tools and equipment to do your job?" For example, a surgeon may tell the operating room staff that it would be helpful to have "PACS" in the operating room to view patient films. Although he or she may have requested this for years, without a formal communication channel, the physician may have become discontent and dissatisfied without the necessary tools and equipment to improve his or her work.

By asking questions about adequate tools and equipment, the hospital is able to be proactive versus reactive to physicians who become discontent. Implementation of critical communication tactics allows physicians to see the hospital's desire to meet their needs, which will build trust and appreciation that the hospital has their best interest at heart.

Physicians would like to have active participation in a newly aligned arrangement. They desire to give input and place emphasis on quality and efficiencies. When physicians are involved in the alignment process, the outcome will be much more successful. The hospital should ensure that the physicians' goals align with the overall organizational goals. This can be accomplished by allowing the physicians to be active participants in the hospital annual strategic planning sessions along with the board of trustees. If the physicians meet their mutually agreed-upon goals, the hospital will meet theirs, which is a win-win situation for the organization.

The aligned groups of physicians want a clear acknowledgment from the hospital that the physicians and their staff (practice administrator, leaders, front- and back-office staff, and nurses) know their business better than what the hospital administration contends to know. A typical alignment failure includes a health system or hospital believing it can run a practice in the same way it runs the hospital. Therefore, one recommendation (and typical arrangement) is for the current practice leadership and management of the practice to stay intact, in some manner, as appropriate.

Adequate Market Share

Physicians desire to participate in any and all market share advancements for both internal and external customers whose needs and expectations drive the design of their products and services. This would include sheer numbers and also percentages accumulated within each primary and secondary market segment, with the goal of increasing exposure and market share percentage. It is essential to know which physicians are driving the volume and where they are sending their business. Involvement of the physicians is critical. Without review, analysis, and discussion with the physicians of physician referral outmigration, it will be difficult to gain a competitive edge.

Further, physicians like to participate in discussions regarding additional services and hours of coverage that affect the go-forward strategy of their practices. When potential decisions will be made about a physician or his or her practice, the hospital should allow the physician an opportunity to have input on the situation. This can be accomplished by a face-to-face meeting to openly discuss the issue at hand. Once all parties have met, reviewed the issues, and made decisions, it is good to take time to confirm what everyone agreed upon and distribute meeting minutes to all attendees. This process provides an opportunity to lay out expectations for both parties and also shows the decision was a collaborative one.

Physicians want to feel comfortable and confident that the hospital leadership has prerequisite knowledge and market awareness, thus enabling the practice to have the best chance for survival in any newly contemplated arrangement. The hospital should recruit a practice management executive to manage the physician practices who can be a leader for both the physician and staff. Physicians want someone who can provide guidance and define a clear vision and strategy.

The practice executive should be someone the physicians will come to respect and trust; someone they know has their best interest at heart but also can have difficult conversations with them, if needed. Physicians want to feel comfortable that the leader has a good decision-making process and that he or she will follow up expediently on needed items.

Therefore, the practice executive needs to communicate well, both verbally and in writing. The practice leader must be able to maintain confidentiality; this will earn trust and respect from the physicians. There must be a good balance from the practice executive that supports both the hospital and physician.

The practice leader must also be a strategic thinker; not only focused on the day-to-day operations but also aware of what is happening in the industry. He or she must be able to transition the physicians to many of the initiatives that are driving healthcare (e.g., electronic health records [EHR], physician quality reporting initiative, ePrescribing, patient-centered medical homes, accountable care organizations). For the hospital to be successful, it is critical for the practice to be successful and to have leaders who are strategic thinkers.

By having a practice leader who is knowledgeable, has good leadership skills, and is a good communicator, the physicians will be comfortable with the leader's ability to keep moving the practice forward in this competitive market.

Continuing Education and Training

Physicians desire enhanced access to education and training, both for themselves and their staff. Continuing medical education (CME) is important for achieving and maintaining credentials and licensure requirements of physicians. The hospital should encourage physician CME that meets professional and state requirements and that is a benefit to hospital-based practices. Hospitals should reimburse physicians for their reasonable and necessary expenses incurred for CME that will be consistent with the IRS guidelines for qualified business travel. Physicians reasonably expect a dollar amount allotted to them each year along with a certain number of days—usually five to 10 work days—to be set aside for CME.

Participation in Managed Care Plans

Collective hospital and physician cooperation has much more bargaining power. A coordinated effort to tackle managed care organizations should be clearly driven by the hospital but be apparent as to its benefit to the physicians and the respective practices. Physician-hospital integration reflects both physician and hospital response to competitive pressures from expanding insurance plans. Alignment allows hospitals and physicians to have more bargaining power and economy of scale with the carriers. Without hospitals, solo physicians/smaller physician groups have little bargaining power with managed care plans. Conversely, hospitals without physicians in the same managed care plans results in patient and physician dissatisfaction, which ultimately reflects poorly on the hospital.

Alignment produces greater efficiency in coordination of managed care. It is easier to pull information and submit it to the carrier collectively. Reviewing utilization and benchmarking is simplified. If both parties fail to reach an agreement, either party can walk away from the network, which would dramatically impact the carriers' demand for their members. If the members are limited on being treated by their physicians due to a breakdown in negotiations, it will have a negative financial impact on the carrier and will also result in member dissatisfaction. This fact validates the benefits of alignment regarding managed care initiatives.

Financial Support and Compensation

Careful and accurate consideration must be given to the go-forward financial impact of any newly aligned arrangement. The physicians must be absolutely confident that there will be an increased financial impact (particularly including their compensation) that results from the alignment consideration. A good place to start is with the physician contract and the bonus incentive plan. Once the physician knows the expectations for the practice/hospital volumes, the practice leader should put action plans in place to help the physicians meet their goals so they see their potential in increasing their compensation.

The hospital should submit monthly financial and variance reports to the physicians that include:

- Physician work relative value unit (wRVU) benchmarks

- Actual wRVU numbers

- Goal on number of visits per month

- Actual visits for the month

It is good for physicians to see their variances. Hospital leadership should also meet with the physicians routinely to discuss the results. When it is time for bonuses to be calculated, there will be no surprises for either side. Further, the practice must be confident that it will benefit from any current or future consideration of accountable care as it is certain to affect the healthcare environment in the next two to five years.

Access to Capital

Physicians need access to additional capital in order to fund current operations, future operations, and new technology (i.e., EHR). A hospital or health system can greatly benefit the physicians in this arrangement through its access to capital funding sources. Typically, this access to capital is due to limitations in cash flow. Supply vendors expect "net-30" terms for payment for goods or services. Employees expect timely paychecks, yet payments from third-party payers average 45 days or more. As a result, physicians need access to capital/loans to keep their practice equipped with current technology and equipment and staffing. Lenders require, at a minimum, current and prior two-year financial statements in order to gauge the credit worthiness of the practice request for loans or capital advances.

Work-Life Balance

Physicians must have peace of mind regarding work-life balance as they con-template an alignment structure. If the alignment model entails transfer of ownership to the hospital, the alignment should represent relief for the physicians from the stresses of owning and managing their practices. Reduction in stress pertains to deriving sources of business, achieving a positive bottom line, increases in malpractice and other insurance challenges, managing staff, and possibly managing other physicians/partners, all of which the hospital will now be responsible.

Summary

Physicians and hospitals have many of the same goals in alignment, although their perspectives differ considerably. They both want to deliver quality patient care; both entities must do so in the most efficient model to maintain stability and achieve profitability in an insecure healthcare environment.

Hospital Perspective

What do hospitals need in physician relationships, and why are they entering alignment initiatives? Hospital leadership has evolved from its prior model, which could be described somewhat like a three-legged stool. Previously, the hospital administrator (now an outdated term) functioned more like an elected coordinating leader than today's CEO, who now bears total responsibility for the organization.

The three legs of the stool representing the balancing influences that worked together to provide patient care as a hospital organization were: the administrator, the physician staff, and the community represented by the governing board. (See Figure 7.1.) The hospital administrator provided 24-hour nursing care, surgical suites, diagnostic equipment, bricks and mortar, and the necessary endless organizational details. The governing board delegated operational responsibility to the administrator while focusing on the hospital's next building fund campaign and other capital initiatives and at the same time maintaining fiduciary responsibility for the hospital for the community. The physicians were independent, seeing patients in their offices, and admitting and attending to their patients in the hospital.

Medicare changed the way physicians practiced and how hospitals provided care. Prior to Medicare, physicians provided most of their care at the hospital because their offices had no word processing, no information systems, no MRIs, no CAT scanners, and only minor laboratory and radiology capabilities. Essentially, all procedures required patients to be hospitalized; therefore, the three-legged stool concept provided a balance of interests. Physicians needed the diagnostic technology, modest compared with today's hospital capabilities, and the 24-hour nursing support for their patients. Hospitals needed physicians to admit patients and to direct patients' care. Each leg of the stool was necessary. At times, however, the

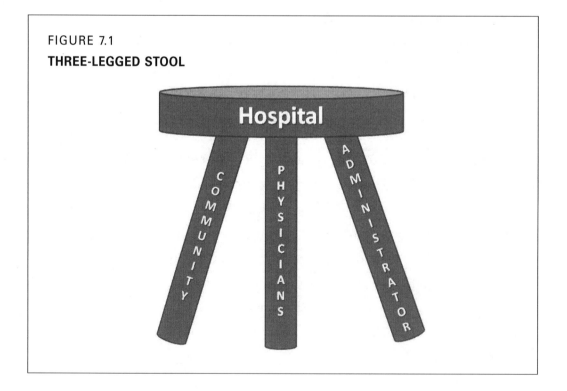

FIGURE 7.1
THREE-LEGGED STOOL

The Healthcare Executive's Guide to Physician-Hospital Alignment

separate legs of the stool had divergent interests due to separate financial needs and no common overreaching factor influencing how they operated or practiced.

Today's hospitals and physicians continue to work to provide quality, cost-effective care. The changes in and demands of the healthcare environment require hospitals and physicians to take another look at the three-legged stool.

The successful hospital CEO views the overall organization in much the same way as a general manager views a sports franchise. The franchise may have the best quarterback in the league, but without protection from the pass rush and receivers to elude the defense and catch the ball, the team cannot win. The general manager does not personally have the skills of the quarterback, the blockers, or the receivers, but he knows what skills are necessary and must assemble a winning team using available resources. The hospital patient care environment is much the same. Without the support of the complete team and the required technology, the best cardiothoracic surgeon, standing alone, would be of little value to the patient. The CEO, in this case, like the general manager, must assemble the best patient care team possible using available resources. Neither the general manager nor the hospital CEO have unlimited resources.

Changes in payment for physician and reimbursement for hospital services are making it necessary for two legs of the stool—physicians and hospitals—to function as one, balancing their individual needs with the overall patient care needs of their service area, and in some instances, far beyond. Couple these reimbursement changes (i.e., providing more care for less payment) with changes made due to federal, state, local, and individual budgetary realities, and the balancing process becomes even more difficult. What, then, do hospitals (CEOs) want and need?

Quality Care

Just as in the days of Florence Nightingale, hospitals want to do no patient harm. A tongue-in-cheek response would be if there were no patients there would be no harm done. However, no risk, no care, and a total disregard for community healthcare needs is unrealistic and irresponsible. A surgeon who has a patient he believes to have appendicitis must determine his future actions. He can perform surgery removing the appendix, exposing the patient to the risks of an untoward reaction to anesthesia, postoperative hospital-acquired infection, a technical surgical error on his part, and/or other bad episodes that can occur within a hospital; or he can make the decision to not intervene. Even to the nonphysician, it is clear that the consequences of not surgically intervening far outweigh the possible surgical risks. CEOs also function in the real world with real risks, real rewards, and real consequences—favorable or unfavorable.

CEOs work through people with responsibility for an organization composed of intertwined systems, each with strengths and weaknesses. The CEO's role is to add to the strengths of the organization while minimizing the weaknesses, and while balancing the needs of the community with the capabilities of the hospital. This leads to the question: what do CEOs want based on the reality of today's hospital environment to meet basic requirements for hospital operation? A hypothetical survey of hospital CEOs would result in a list of wants that include:

- Competent physicians in specialties required to provide patient care for services provided by the hospital

- Competent physicians for the community's need for non-hospital services

- An organized quality-focused medical staff

- Competent nursing staff and other allied health staff organized to support patient care services provided by the hospital

- Physical plant and diagnostic equipment necessary to provide care for services provided by the hospital

- An information system that meets both clinical and financial needs for the hospitals and physicians

- Patient volumes necessary for efficient and quality hospital operation

- Financial results with a margin adequate to provide current services and planning for future required services as well as improvement of current services

As hospitals have evolved, CEOs have used different approaches to acquire the items on this list. Remember the three-legged stool? During a much different time with different physician attitudes, physician education and capabilities, financial payment, available diagnostic capabilities, and patient and community expectations, the CEO's role was also much different. In the past, physicians typically moved into a town and applied for privileges by joining an existing physician practice. The hospital did not feel the need to provide financial assistance. Hospital services evolved over time based on the overall mix of physicians in a given discipline on the hospital's medical staff. Other than the physicians' office practices, all community healthcare was centered at the hospital. When more than one hospital served a community, typically physicians would serve on more than one medical staff and hospitals, in general, would focus on different specialties. One hospital would focus on obstetrics while another would focus on orthopedics, and the like. State regulatory Certificate of Need requirements for capital expenditures and new services also limited competition among hospitals. Nonprofit hospitals were the norm.

There have been major improvements to types of services offered due to changes as a result of physicians and hospitals being better prepared and equipped to provide improved outcomes for more patient diagnoses. It has been some time since patients surviving the initial assault of a myocardial infarction were given morphine, oxygen, and bed rest, and either survived or expired. Today, cardiac catheterization capability and other interventions are taken for granted; the cardiologist is far more than a "watch and wait" practitioner. The education and training of physicians and the advent of new technology and procedural equipment has changed how coronary disease is treated, for example, as well as patient outcomes. For countless patients, artificial joint replacement surgery and restoration of mobility has made reliance on crutches and wheelchairs a thing of the past. As physician and hospital capabilities have advanced, so has the complexity of hospital operations.

Satisfactory Margins

What events led to today's increasing rate of change in patient services provided? The watershed event was the creation of Medicare and Medicaid in 1966. Medicare coverage expanded in 1972 with coverage for the disabled and the addition of kidney dialysis. Medicare expanded again in 2003 with the addition of payment for outpatient drugs. Prior to Medicare, families pooled finances to pay medical and hospital bills for aging family members when the patient did not have the necessary resources, or relied on charity from their physician and hospital. Before Medicaid, the medically indigent did not receive care or also relied on physician and hospital charity. With the advent of Medicare and Medicaid, hospitals were now paid for the cost of caring for many patients that, before, would have been provided care for no payment. At the same time, the advancement of technology to further healthcare exploded and part of the cost of acquiring new technology was now transferred to the government.

The entry of investor-owned hospital companies into the market such as National Medical Enterprises (now Tenet) in 1967 and Hospital Corporation of America (now HCAHealthcare) in 1968, changed how hospitals operate. Hospitals are run more like businesses than charitable organizations, and competition among hospitals is overt and planned. Hospitals are no longer passively working with physicians choosing to apply for privileges. Successful nonprofit and investor-owned hospitals are operated in much the same way. All hospitals need to produce an adequate financial operating margin to survive. The investor-owned participants expect value appreciation. A quote by Sister Irene Kraus of the Daughters of

Charity National Health Care System, "No Margin, No Mission," stated the obvious for the nonprofit sector.[1]

Market Share

The Health Maintenance Act of 1973 greatly expanded managed care and created more change. Now the hospital's market share influenced the rates the hospitals were paid. Capturing market share became the CEO's priority. CEOs focused on patient volumes while other administrative staff members focused on the internal hospital operations. Physicians, like hospitals, were paid negotiated rates (managed care lingo for "less payment"). Physicians and hospitals formed physician hospital organizations to be better prepared to negotiate with the managed care (insurance) companies. Some contracts included financial risk in the form of patient capitation payments and some contracts included risk based on patient outcomes. It became obvious that the future combined financial viability of the physician's practice and the hospital depended on the individual success of each. The two were tied together.

The Emergency Medical Treatment and Active Labor Act of 1986 (EMTALA) increased the necessity for hospital CEOs to access the capability and availability of medical staff members in regard to patients coming to the emergency department for care. Emergency department physician-on-call coverage became even more important. Financial penalties would result if a patient was transferred from a hospital emergency department to another hospital if the first hospital could have appropriately cared for the transferred patient. CEOs, if not already doing so, were focusing on the breadth and depth of the hospital medical staff. The Patient

Safety and Quality Improvement Act of 2005 is another example of legislation requiring hospitals and physicians to work together as a team in order to protect the patient as optimally as possible.

Physician Collaboration

As stated earlier in the chapter, alignment is absolutely necessary today as hospitals and physicians must be consistently working toward a win-win conclusion to ensure future success. The Patient Protection and Affordable Care Act of 2010 and the Accountable Care Organization (ACO) reimbursement methodology's anticipated impact on physicians and hospitals has made it necessary for physicians and hospitals to work more like a coordinated team than separate entities. The hospital CEO, like the general manager of the sports franchise, and physician stakeholders, like the superstars on the team, must work closely together. Their interests are financially and conceptually aligned. The new risk-reward sharing ACO reimbursement methodology, although in the demonstration phase and only found in very large provider organizations, is an additional stimulus for hospitals and physicians to work together as a true team.

The three-legged stool (community represented by the governing board, the hospital administrator, and the physician staff) that provided patient care as a hospital organization has evolved to today's teeter-totter with community healthcare needs and expectations on one side and the hospital organization and its physician staff on the other. (See Figure 7.2.) The CEO's (previously called the administrator) role is to lead the healthcare organization to keep this teeter-totter in balance.

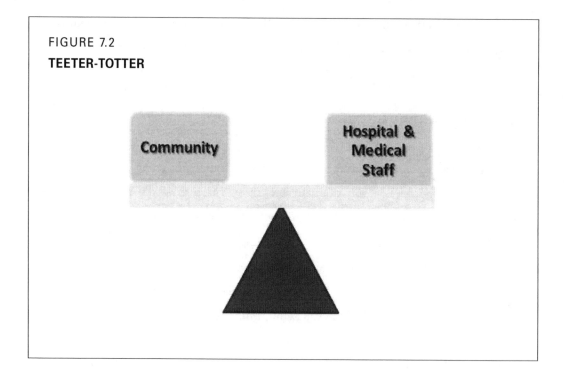

FIGURE 7.2

TEETER-TOTTER

Partnership Against the Competition

In alignment strategies, hospitals want physicians to be attentive to improving and growing market share, which serves the needs of both parties. Although pursuit of market share growth (i.e., attempting to increase volumes and numbers) is often viewed as offensive, this strategy can be considered a defensive approach to protect the loss of patients to competitors and other hospitals that desire to increase their market share in your market area. Realistically, maintaining and increasing your presence in more locations and with more technology is a matter of protecting (or defending) your organization against others who would invade your market position.

Similarly, hospitals must remain competitive from a cost perspective. The concept is that more coverage, more specialists, more primary physician care, more procedures, and more surgeries would affect economies of scale and reduce the overall cost of services. The reality is that the hospital is simply looking to maintain and improve its bottom line. Very similar to market share concerns is the hospital's desire to maintain its positive image and name recognition within the community. Having combined forces and synchronized efforts with its community physicians, the hospital has a better opportunity for increased favorable opinion by the community.

Positioning for the ACO Criteria

Another significant need of the hospital because of the current healthcare environment is that of positioning. Hospitals must synchronize and align with physicians to demonstrate urgent and specific readiness for ACOs and other integrated clinical affiliations. Those paying attention to accountable care and integrated clinical affiliations are in the best position for achieving success— whether success is defined in clinical or financial terms. Alignment can only help further this initiative. Alignment should be viewed as a progressive action toward improving quality and achieving better medical/clinical outcomes.

From a hospital's perspective, influencing collaboration between the physicians and the hospital is also seen as a buffer to the current legal and regulatory challenges affecting the healthcare environment. Federal regulations regarding integrated care provide safe harbors for hospitals and physicians against violations from federal regulations such as anti-kickback and antitrust legislation.

Decreased HCIT Costs and Improved Efficiencies

Healthcare information technology (HCIT) is a significant consideration in any operation. With the move towards alignment, the perceived and desired outcome should be decreased costs and increased efficiencies through the hospital and physicians working together on IT platforms and sharing information (within legal parameters). HCIT can play a major role in the success of the combined operation. When all providers work on the same system/platform, they can reduce overall cost of delivery by providing better information throughout their organization. This saves time, which in effect saves money; better efficiencies hold down costs and result in improved outcomes for the patients.

The Continual Process—Dealing With Reality

Having everything on the "want list" is not a recipe for success; neither is it possible nor acceptable simply to have every item on the list. Puzzle pieces do not create a picture by themselves. The separate items on a CEO's want list by themselves—even when each item is present—are of limited value. Their value lies in how the pieces are coordinated and utilized. Today's healthcare arena calls for the most efficient use of resources through streamlined alignment initiatives with physicians. No longer are hospitals merely competing with each other to garner the greatest market share, they are competing for survival of the fittest.

Today, hospitals need a team comprising all stakeholders (i.e., all members of the medical staff, hospital employees, the hospital board of trustees, and contracted hospital departments), who are all focused on delivering the best patient care at the lowest possible cost in the most appropriate setting while also planning for providing human and financial resources in the future. Does this sound reasonable? It is! It is not, however, an easy task. Regarding hospital management, Peter Drucker said, "The hospital is altogether the most complex human organization ever devised."[2] The challenges are great and, for the community, success is mandatory.

The term best describing the hospital's process to meet this challenge is *continuous active alignment*. In this context, continuous active alignment is a series of events or steps with no reversals, by involved, energetic—rather than speculative—individuals with a common understanding of the purposes and goals of the organization. The hospital must know what it wishes to accomplish, the required "puzzle pieces," the required and available financial resources, the anticipated time requirements, and each step necessary to create the desired outcome (picture) using the puzzle pieces. So, where do we begin?

For our purposes, we will assume the hospital is a non-teaching, community urban acute-care medical-surgical facility. Again, picture the teeter-totter diagram. The hospital is not alone on the teeter-totter. To achieve balance, the current and projected characteristics of the community must be identified as well as current and projected healthcare needs based on these characteristics and the current status of the hospital and medical staff capabilities. Determining unmet community need is an arduous and soul-searching endeavor. There are differences in opinion as to how community need is determined; services pro-vided, necessary patient outmigration for specific care, availability of after hours care, and the like are all issues to be reconciled. We will assume community need has been established.

Let us begin with the physician stakeholders. Physician stakeholders come to the healthcare team as a product of diverse cultures; education and training; differing years of experience, capabilities, and life experiences; and differing visions of what being a physician should be, as well as financial expectations. Some physician stakeholders are natural leaders and have a strong desire to be in charge, while others prefer more of a passive role. Some may have been in the community for many years arriving with no outside assistance; others may have joined other physicians; some may have been recruited on short-term income guarantee arrangements; and others may be employed. With this in mind, what are the hospital's physician needs? Where do we start?

For the concept of continuous active alignment to be of benefit, we must have a starting point. The hospital's starting point is the hospital's physician "depth and breadth chart." (See Figure 7.3.) The exercise of creating the physician depth and breadth chart is a good use of the CEO's time. This cannot be accomplished in a vacuum and requires candid input from current physicians, hospital professional staff and, in some cases, outside physician community-need consultants. Physician needs can be determined, much like determining what a sports team needs to be competitive and to win, both done through charting. The continuous active alignment process that began with determining community need and comparing the need with the physician depth and breadth chart is now under way. We can now address the question: what do hospitals want and need? Earlier we listed a CEO want list. All line items on that listing are needed for the hospital's long-term success. What is needed to organize the puzzle pieces completes the answer to the question.

FIGURE 7.3

COMMUNITY HOSPITAL DEPTH & BREADTH CHART

SPECIALTY	CURRENT	NEED	PLAN	NOTES
Fam Med	12	10		
IM	10	12	2	
Peds				
Cardiology	6	8	2	invasive
Gastro	4	4		
Neurology	2	3	1	
OB-GYN	8	8		
Critical Care	3	4	1	
GenSurg	4	4		
Ortho	6	8	2	Sports
Urology	6	8	2	Robotic
Hospitalist	6	0	6	New
More	X	X	X	

Note: Need based on third-party physician needs analysis and CEO/medical leadership dialogue.

An abundance of material is written on physician-hospital alignment. Alignment frameworks include: professional service agreements, employment agreements, modified employment agreements ("employment lite"), clinically integrated networks, physician practice purchase agreements, and others. These agreements between physicians and hospitals are written for the purpose of creating a framework to align the interests of the physicians and the hospital in order for them to better work together to address the challenges of meeting community healthcare needs in today's healthcare environment.

Candid professional dialogue between the physicians—regardless of their agreement—and the hospital is necessary for the physician depth and breadth chart to be of value. The patient population and the population's healthcare basic needs have been identified. Statistically, the required raw number for each type of physician for the identified population's needs is available. The candid professional dialogue enables the hospital to adjust the "statistical physician numbers" and complete the physician depth and breadth chart based on the real world of the varying characteristics of physician stakeholders previously mentioned.

The nuances of each chart entry are of critical importance. As an example, statistical information is available on the predicted occurrence of most disease entities for a given defined population, your service area. What should the hospital and physician capabilities be? Open heart surgery is not performed in all hospitals but there will be a need for open heart surgery for some people in every service area. Organ transplant capability is another example. A clear understanding of the hospital's role in the overall delivery of care is a minimum need. Again, this calls for candid professional dialogue.

For example, after determining that care for individuals in the area of urology is one of the needs the hospital should provide, the current capability status must be addressed. How many urologists are required to meet service-area patient needs?

Raw numbers do not work without the accompanying physician-hospital dialogue. For the teeter-totter to be in balance, the total physician and hospital capabilities must be in balance with community healthcare needs. What if all the urologists on the hospital staff are de facto retired and no longer providing surgery, preferring a 100% office practice? Although they may be aligned with the hospital using the hospital's diagnostic services, are they meeting the hospital's needs? Their patients that require surgery are being cared for at another hospital. Where would they be on the physician depth and breadth chart? This is a clearly identified need that must be satisfied for the teeter-totter to be in balance. In this instance, to meet the healthcare needs of the community, the CEO, like the sports team general manger, must add the required number of urologists with the appropriate education and training. If, however, the required number of urologists with the necessary education, training, and interests are present, the CEO focuses on the continuous active alignment of this capability.

Summary

The simplistic examples used in this chapter do not capture the true complexity of balancing the needs of the community with the capabilities (and needs) of the physicians and the hospital. They do, however, illustrate how to identify physician-hospital alignment needs. Physicians and hospitals are being pushed together, some reluctantly, by the changes outlined here. Physicians and hospitals looking forward understand both physicians and hospitals will continue to be expected to do more with less. Physicians and hospitals committed to the continuous active alignment methodology will be better prepared to meet the healthcare needs of their community and keep the teeter-totter in balance.

The hospital "want" list and "need" list are the same. How to achieve the want list and how to organize the want list "pieces" to become a picture of a hospital providing quality cost-effective care, balancing its needs as an organization with the patient care needs of the community, differentiates the great provider organizations from all others. Using the tools available to the hospital today, employing an active continuous alignment process, a hospital and medical staff working as one can be a great provider.

REFERENCES

1. No Margin, No Mission: Flying Nuns and Sister Irene Kraus. Accessed 9/12/2012 at *http://blog. teletracking.com/bid/129616/No-Margin-No-Mission-Flying-Nuns-and-Sister-Irene-Kraus.*

2. Drucker, Peter. *Managing in the Next Society* (Burlington, MA: Elsevier Ltd, 2002). Accessed 9/12/2012 at *http://books.google.com/books?id=wAFdkE3GFpoC&lpg=PT165&ots=CT8lpCbpqE& dq=the%20hospital.*

Compensation Strategies

Chapter 4 introduced us to the three levels of integration (limited, moderate, and full) and outlined the basic tenets of the various alignment models that fall within each level. A key component within each alignment strategy is the compensation physicians receive for their services. Where these physicians fall on the integration continuum is the ultimate determinant of the framework that will make up their compensation. As the strategy increases in complexity, the physicians become more financially tethered to the other parties in the mix, and their payment methodologies follow suit. The main thrust of this chapter is to explore the varying compensation frameworks within each alignment strategy. As you will notice, compensation models vary along alignment models as well as integration levels.

Limited Integration Strategies

Managed care networks

Physicians that belong to managed care networks, such as independent practice associations (IPA) or physician hospital organizations (PHO), realize very little impact in their pay from participation. Oftentimes, belonging to a managed care network impacts a practice's payer contracts, in that they are no longer contracting independently, but potentially as part of the managed care network. With this in mind, the key way that compensation is affected is when there is a positive change in payer contracts. Meaning, if participation in the IPA or PHO can lead to better reimbursement, this ultimately impacts physician compensation by increasing it, assuming all other factors (e.g., overhead) remain unchanged.

Also, if these networks are used as platforms for accountable care organization (ACO) development, providers may realize an increase in compensation from incentive distribution. An example of this is a clinically integrated network that is formed by a health system, which includes the health system's employed physicians as well as a host of private practice physicians who are willing to be active participants in the ACO. Based on the scope of the ACO and the individual physician performance, physicians could receive distributions that would supplement their income. Currently, distributions from an ACO or ACO-like entity tend to be in addition to fee-for-service reimbursement, not a replacement of fee-for-service reimbursement. Thus, the ACO distributions represent a new source of funding.

In all other cases, however, compensation remains unaffected on account of this strategy. Thus, if anything, when integrating via IPAs or PHOs, there may potentially be some incremental increases in reimbursement as part of payer contracting changes, but these alone would not necessarily be paradigm shifting and may not have any impact on the underlying compensation plan within the respective private groups (or hospital-employed groups).

Call coverage stipends

Unlike the aforementioned scenario, call coverage stipends offer providers an additional stream of revenue. The compensation from this strategy can potentially result in substantial economic benefits to physicians that provide a large amount of coverage. However, before we continue our discussion on payment models, it is important to differentiate between the two types of physician call coverage: restricted and unrestricted. Unrestricted call coverage entails physicians responding to inquiries (or pages) within a set period of time or based on degree of trauma. The physicians don't have to be on-site, just on call. Conversely, physicians providing restricted call coverage have to be on-site at the hospital for the duration of their coverage. There is added burden associated with restricted call coverage because the physician cannot engage in other revenue-generating cases (clinic time, elective surgeries, etc.) and must actually remain physically present at the hospital, often having to sleep at the hospital. Because of this added burden and higher opportunity cost (i.e., cannot generate other revenue as one can when providing unrestricted call) associated with restricted call coverage, the compensation levels are generally higher for this arrangement than for unrestricted call.

Despite the overall burdens associated with being on-call, there are three main types of burdens that physicians face when responding to unassigned calls, which usually have a direct impact on the compensation received. They are:

- Financial burden

- Personal burden

- Risk/liability

Financial burden

In many, if not most, call compensation programs, the primary driver for the physicians desiring compensation is the financial burden associated with providing call coverage. Many hospitals have a high population of indigent care patients (self-pay) that utilize the emergency department (ED) as their healthcare provider. This results in the physicians on the hospitals' medical staffs that participate in the ED call rotation providing a significant amount of services but receiving little, if any, remuneration. Due to the response requirements of providing unassigned call coverage, physicians, at times, have to cancel clinics or delay surgical cases that offer better (i.e., higher) reimbursement in order to see unassigned patients in the ED or work surgical cases on indigent patients. Many of the unassigned patients that require care from the on-call physicians need some level of follow-up care. Thus, these patients then see the physicians in their outpatient setting, again presenting another opportunity in which the physician provides services for little remuneration.

The financial burden of unassigned call coverage is real but, of course, varies by location. Geographical settings that have a very poor payer mix often need to pay for call or employ the most needed physicians in order to remain viable. Hospitals where the payer mix is more favorable typically are not as inclined to pay for call.

Personal burden

The impact of call on quality of life is a key factor, especially for the population of younger physicians. Unrestricted call coverage requires physicians to modify their personal lives to enable them to be responsive to the hospital when on call. This can take the form of being within 30 minutes of the hospital when on call, not consuming alcohol, and not taking part in other activities that could keep the physicians from being able to deliver quality patient care. Many calls from the hospital occur in the evenings, interrupting the time physicians spend with their families as well as their sleep habits.

This burden can be exacerbated by the specialty and the number of physicians in the call rotation. Certain specialties, such as general surgery and orthopedic surgery, typically have a much higher call load (i.e., a greater number of telephone consults and required presentations to the ED) and, therefore, experience a more significant personal burden. If a low number of physicians within a specialty are sharing the call coverage duties, the result can be an added burden due to the sheer number of days on call.

Often, the number of telephone consultations a physician is required to perform can be just as burdensome as having to physically come into the ED during a period of call coverage. These telephone consultations are rarely, if ever, billable.

Risk/liability

Unassigned call coverage often requires physicians to perform procedures or provide medical consultation to patients who have not historically had the proper medical care or have multiple medical conditions that complicate the rendering of proper medical care. Often, the physician has to provide services to a patient with whom the physician is not familiar. All of these factors increase the potential for medical errors/complications, and increase the potential for medical malpractice lawsuits. This then increases the cost of professional liability insurance the physician is required to carry.

Physicians also risk harming their own patients when on call. Being on call may require physicians to provide medical services in the middle of the night. Most often, the physician is holding clinic or has scheduled procedures for the following day. If a physician receives little sleep the night before, it can potentially result in medical errors and places the physician at an increased level of malpractice risk.

In many instances, a hospital's medical staff bylaws or a physician's employment agreement will require a baseline level of call coverage. For example, it may require each physician to provide five days of on-call coverage per month. If this is the case, it is typical for only excess calls to be compensated.

A number of different payment methodologies for call coverage exist within the industry. Here is an explanation of the following four potential compensation alternatives:

- Stipend model

- Hybrid model (stipend plus fee-for-service)

- Fee-for-service model

- Deferred compensation model

Stipend model

In this model, the hospital pays a negotiated fair market value compensation for service line call coverage. While there are several variations of the stipend model, a stipend based on a daily rate (24 hours) is the most common method for on-call services due to the ease of calculating the compensation amount and the fact that it takes into consideration the overall burden of performing call duties. More often than not, the daily stipend model entails a flat fee that is established prior to the work being completed, based upon industry comparisons and other more "standard" data. It is not derived from any specific basis of actual work performed.

In addition to a daily stipend, the stipend model can be applied to other situations such as a per-response or per-beeper payment for every telephone consult and visit to the ED. However, data regarding these metrics must be retained in order to apply the model in this manner. Moreover, payment based upon such criteria could become tedious and argumentative (e.g., how many beeps? How many calls? How many trips to the ED?) Based on industry data, the stipend model still appears to be the most prevalent form of compensation for physicians performing ED call and, frankly, is the simplest method to calculate. Keep in mind that does not mean it is the best payment method.

Fee-for-service model

The fee-for-service model does not include a daily stipend. Rather, it only provides physicians fee-for-service payment for uninsured patients, including those with no insurance and those who are self-pay. Payments to the physicians can be based on the actual current procedural terminology codes charged, and reimbursement is typically at Medicare rates (or slightly higher). Alternatively, reimbursement may be based on a fixed amount per physician work relative value unit (wRVU). A third alternative is to have a flat fee for various services performed for uninsured patients.

The fee-for-service model requires a trusting working relationship between the hospital and the physicians. To receive payment, physicians are required to share some portion of their financials with the hospital (at the very least, that information related to uninsured patients).

Hybrid model

The hybrid model provides the physicians with both a stipend and remuneration for the uncompensated care they provide. The stipend is typically a fixed, daily total and less than that what traditionally be offered under a straight stipend model. This is because it is meant only to compensate the physicians for the personal burden they assume as a result of being on call.

In addition to the stipend, the physicians also receive compensation for the uninsured patients (strictly self-pay) they see, for whom they would normally not receive any reimbursement. This additional compensation is meant to compensate the physicians for the financial burden they assume when taking call. The fee-for-service reimbursement is based on the work actually performed by the physician (as opposed to a set rate), and is normally driven by the current Medicare fee schedule. Some hospitals choose to pay a premium on Medicare rates, but typically this is not more than 5%–10%.

Deferred compensation model

As remuneration for call coverage, deferred compensation is provided to the physician vis-à-vis their individual investment portfolio or retirement fund. In this structure, the hospital provides a deferred *contribution* rather than a deferred *benefit*; that is, the hospital does not guarantee any specific amount will be available to the physician after the vesting period. Rather, the hospital agrees to deposit a set monetary value in the physician's investment account, and that value is held at risk for gains or losses, similar to any other market-based investment.

In the deferred compensation model, the hospital provides a deposit (at a constant amount) to each physician for every 24-hour shift the physician completes unassigned call coverage. These deposits are credited to a physician's account on a quarterly basis for services provided in each calendar quarter. No compensation is paid for any services if the physician has not submitted medical record documentation as required by the hospital. The money is held in an investment account for a vesting period, often a five-year period, after which it is accessible to the physicians.

This model is beneficial to the hospital because the hospital does not have to pay physicians immediately for the services they perform while on call, keeping a financial tie with physicians for a set amount of time (often five years). Using a market-based investment also has a potential upside for the physicians as their investment could increase at a high rate of return.

When making decisions relative to the actual amount of compensation to provide to physicians, there are several methods for arriving at the most appropriate rate. Market and benchmark data such as the Sullivan, Cotter and Associates, Inc. (SCA) *Physician On-Call Pay Survey Report* and the Medical Group Management Association (MGMA) *Medical Directorship and On-Call Compensation Survey*, can serve as primary references for establishing payment rates. In addition to this data, further analysis should be performed that quantitatively assesses the burden associated with providing call coverage so that the compensation can be tailored to the respective burden.

Medical directorships

The compensation model for physicians who engage in medical directorships or other administrative services typically consists of a market-based hourly rate at its foundation. Medical directors are contracted by hospitals to provide administrative and management oversight via agreements that are separate from hospital employment compensation contracts (in some cases, the medical directorship can be embedded in the employment agreement). As noted, these services are compensated on an hourly basis. This arrangement usually entails three factors:

1. Establishing a set hourly rate

2. Defining the number of expected hours

3. Compensating medical directors only for work actually performed

A best practice for physicians who also fulfill medical director roles is to document all hours worked and all services provided to realize an appropriate level of remuneration. This may be done on a timesheet and should require appropriate approvals by the hospital. As is the case with all compensation structures, the rate for medical director and other administrative services should be at fair market value (FMV) and commercially reasonable.

Best practice is to compensate for said services on an hourly basis; however, it is worth noting that in some instances, an attestation process is used. In an attestation arrangement, the medical director's pay is a monthly stipend. For example, if compensation for this position is $24,000 annually, this would come to a monthly stipend of $2,000. The physician then provides certification that he or she is performing all necessary duties. In some cases, the provider may submit a written report outlining what he or she has accomplished along with the certification as additional documentation of the work performed. Although the hourly rate process is cleaner, in some instances, due to the nature of the work (i.e., it is hard to separate the medical director's tasks from all other duties), the attestation process is appropriate.

In determining the FMV limitations on the total compensation that can be provided to the physicians that also act as medical directors, one important component is the time spent performing these services. In most instances, payment is based solely on documented hours worked. Therefore, it is imperative for the medical director to document time spent performing the necessary administrative services (it is recommended this be completed on a weekly basis). The hospital can then affirm the time spent and compensate the physician based on his or her individual number of recorded hours.

Early in the process, administrators must determine the number of hours that may be required for medical directors to perform the services of their agreement. To establish values for these hours, industry and benchmark data can be used. For example, the MGMA *Medical Directorship and On-Call Compensation Survey* can provide values for hours spent per week on directorship duties for applicable specialties.

To determine the appropriate compensation, data from industry benchmarking surveys, including MGMA and SCA, can be used. In addition, Integrated Healthcare Strategies provides data that often proves useful for medical directorships as it is one of very few medical directorship-specific surveys currently published. It is important to note that clinical compensation rates may not be appropriate for medical directorship duties. As the skill, risk, effort, judgment, and revenue generation is different between clinical and administrative duties, it may warrant a differentiation in value. Further, the position in question should be compensated based on its needs and not necessarily on the specialty of the physician fulfilling the position. As an example, if a pediatric surgeon is fulfilling a director of quality role, it would not necessarily be appropriate to compensate this position at a pediatric surgeon's compensation level. What would be most appropriate is to understand the clinical qualifications necessary to fulfill the director of quality role and the typical compensation in the market for these positions and then establish the compensation level accordingly.

Once the rate and number of required hours have been established, it is recommended that the hospital establish a compensation cap using those two values. The hospital must determine the appropriate level of compensation as well as the level of commitment (in terms of hours) based on its specific situation and need. It is recommended that conservatism be applied when determining the time and compensation so as to ensure that the medical directors will be compensated only for the work they actually perform.

Recruitment/incubation

Recruitment/incubation models involve the local hospital providing support for the recruitment and ramp-up of a physician. In recruitment, the support provided by the hospital is simply a payment to the practice to cover any gap between revenue generated and certain overhead (e.g., physician compensation, benefits, and incremental overhead) for a certain period of time. Incubation is the same scenario, but the new physician is fully employed by the hospital for a set period of time wherein the hospital incurs the loss associated with recruitment and ramp-up. With the recruitment/incubation strategy, the benefit to the existing practice physicians is that their compensation is not as impacted by bringing on a new provider. Depending on the specialty and ramp-up period, this can be substantial. The impact on compensation within recruitment/incubation arrangements can best be described using the following example.

There is a need for a new oncologist at the local clinic, ABC Clinic. The starting salary is $300,000. The potential new oncologist is joining a practice with 10 physicians. When all of the incremental costs are considered, it is going to cost ABC Clinic $500,000 per year to support this new oncologist from a cost standpoint. The new oncologist is not taking over an existing practice, thus volume must be developed from scratch. In the first year, only $200,000 in collections is expected (resulting in a $300,000 deficit). In the second year, $400,000 in collections is expected (yielding a $100,000 deficit). Instead of incurring this cost within ABC Clinic (i.e., decreasing the total compensation pool by $300,000 in year one and $100,000 in year two, a total of $40,000 per physician), ABC Clinic partners with a hospital via an income guarantee. The hospital then guarantees the required costs of $500,000 per year, so long as the physician remains in the community for a total of five years. Thus, it keeps the existing providers secure during recruitment.

Moderate Integration Strategies

As we move up one level of integration, the elements of the relationships found at this level are more intricate than what we discussed in the previous section.

Accordingly, the strategies at play are also more complex in nature. Compared to limited integration, moderately integrated parties are more aligned systematically and financially.

Management services organization

For those physicians that decide to participate in a management services organization (MSO) with a hospital, both parties may realize an additional stream of revenue. This strategy connects a portion of the hospital's income to the physicians' business successes. As discussed in Chapter 4, when exploring the formation of an MSO, hospitals and physicians may join to form a new entity, NewCo, LLC. When physicians provide their management or administrative services through this new entity, the hospital pays NewCo, LLC, a fair market management fee in exchange for these services. This fee may either be a fixed monthly amount or percentage of revenues from these specific services. Sometimes, these physicians may have a performance incentive component to their compensation. The compensation in this case is for *real services*. The benefit to the practice and to the physicians would only be realized if they are able to effectively provide the services so as to realize a margin. Thus, the margin is the real benefit.

Equity model assimilation

Equity model assimilation is another strategy that moderately integrates all those involved. When these parties become connected through legal arrangements, they gain the ability to jointly establish better marketing schemes, ancillary development, and payer contracts. Thus, the parties can potentially realize a profit on account of the improvements in payer contracts and other efficiencies.

The key benefits for engaging in this model include:

- Partner physicians of the practice realize up-front monies when the equity partner buys in

- On an ongoing basis, the practice can benefit through higher revenues from participating in the new equity partner's payer contracts and other resources, which ends up adding to the bottom line

Example: A large multi-specialty group has a desire for some level of alignment with a health system, but does not desire full employment. Discussions were initially held with the local hospital, but an agreement on a transaction could not be reached. The practice then reached out to a much larger health system in the state to explore its options. The two entities agreed to an equity model transaction, wherein the health system would purchase a share of the practice. The transaction resulted in an up-front payment to shareholder physicians, allowing them to cash out on a portion of their equity. The practice also benefits from access to a large pool of resources and better payer contracts, impacting future income levels while maintaining its autonomy. The health system benefits from its reach into a new market and overall expansion of other initiatives (ACO formation, insurance products, etc.).

Clinical co-management/service line management

The final form of moderate integration is the clinical co-management/service line management strategy. Clinical co-management and service line management models have many similarities, with the key difference being the emphasis on call coverage and the emphasis on incentives. Service line management agreements tend to have a strong focus on call coverage and a lesser focus on incentive dollars (though these may well exist), wherein clinical co-management models do not typically include payment for call coverage and are more focused on the potential incentive dollars.

In terms of potential compensation, the clinical co-management model includes two components. The first is the base fee, which represents between 50%–70% of the total potential compensation. It is largely tied to the hours worked by the physicians in pursuing the clinical co-management model. This compensation can be paid on an hourly basis, based on hours worked, or on a more consistent basis, with regular attestation by the physicians that the work is being performed. The remaining compensation is tied to the incentives within the clinical co-management agreement. In most cases, the incentive portion is tied to a series of predetermined payment amounts contingent on achievement of specific, objectively measurable program development; quality improvement; and efficiency goals. The key here is that any remuneration generated by physicians is tied to real work and real achievements. Thus, the physicians must be actively involved in management to benefit from the base fee and, likely, only involvement in day-to-day management will render the success needed to realize the performance incentives.

Service line management agreements are intended to reward physicians for their efforts in developing, managing, and improving the quality and efficiency of a particular hospital service line. A contract relationship will exist between the two entities, defining the relationship and any compensation that will result. In most cases, the compensation is tied to specific services the physicians will provide as well as some compensation associated with the achievement of certain outcomes.

The most common services included in a service line management agreement are call coverage, administrative and clinical services, oversight of the entire hospital departmental specialty services, and then performance incentives (typically tied to both quality outcomes and shared savings).

The administrative and clinical oversight services included tend to be more broadly defined than a basic medical director role, giving the physician(s) more responsibility over various facets of the overall service line. While this can entail more compensation, it also requires more time spent by the physician(s) in terms of performing the administrative and clinical oversight services.

The call coverage tends to take on compensation similar to other call pay arrangements, wherein it can be paid via a daily stipend, fee-for-service, or some hybrid methodology. Often, this pay is implicit to the determined compensation for the service line management agreement, thus not entailing a separate, distinctive amount of pay for call. Hospitals prefer this so they can camouflage this commitment (thereby not setting a precedent to have to pay other specialists).

Performance incentives vary greatly both in form and amount. In most cases, they are focused on quality initiatives (infection rate, readmissions, etc.), patient satisfaction, and cost control (implant costs, etc.). Each year, a scorecard is developed that outlines the areas of focus for that year and how each will be measured and scored. In most cases, the incentive is only paid annually or semi-annually at most. With most service line management agreements, the performance incentives are of lesser focus than the other two components.

Example: A local hospital wants to expand its orthopedic surgery service line. The hospital reaches out to an existing physician professional corporation that specializes in orthopedic services (sports medicine and hand and spine injuries). The hospital contracts with this existing practice via a clinical co-management agreement. This results in the development of a management committee comprised of representatives from both the practice and the hospital providing oversight of orthopedic services. The hospital remunerates the practice with a flat fee for administrative time (for example, $175 per hour) and a contingent fee for achieving performance-based incentive criteria.

Example: An OB-GYN practice of seven physicians is located in a one-hospital town that represents the majority, but not all, of the OB-GYN providers. The local hospital is interested in developing a laborist program and contacted the practice. An independent third party was engaged to review the situation and provide a valuation of the proposed services. The practice already has one physician in the hospital each day managing unassigned call (when they are on call) and taking care of clinic patients. Taking on the laborist role has minimal operational impact, due to the amount of time the physician on call is already in the hospital, but provides another revenue stream. The hospital benefits in this instance as it adds formality to the protocols associated with treating unassigned and emergent OB-GYN patients, which was not necessarily the case when there was simply a basic unassigned call rotation.

Full Integration Strategies

When integration is at its fullest form, (an employment contract or a professional services agreement [PSA]) a significant portion of the physicians' remuneration becomes reliant on the compensation model(s) in place.

Professional services agreements

The PSA, or "employment lite" model, offers three distinct financial arrangements with an additional option for hybrid arrangements. Accordingly, the compensation frameworks to be discussed vary based on the type of arrangement. Compensation structures for hybrid arrangements are subject to the components of the strategy.

Global payment PSA

Under the global payment PSA model, physicians and mid-level providers continue to be employed by the practice but are contracted by the hospital to provide medical/specialty services (i.e., professional services only) on an exclusive basis. Exclusive does not mean that the providers are prohibited from practicing at other hospitals. Rather, it entails that all professional fees generated by these providers—including those generated at other hospitals—will be part of the PSA and its derivative global payment.

The goal of the PSA is to promote a stabilized alignment relationship between the practice and the selected hospital. The PSA will allow the practice to realize improved total "revenue," which will ultimately result in stabilized/improved bottom line compensation for the physicians, yet all the while maintaining total payments within FMV and commercial reasonableness parameters.

Within a global PSA, the practice continues to be responsible for all operating expenses, post-PSA. In return, the practice receives a global payment from the selected hospital partner to cover these expenses (both practice overhead and physician-related expenses). This is in lieu of the practice billing and collecting professional fees. The global payment can be a fixed amount paid on a monthly basis. A preferred alternative, however, is to build the global payment plus incentive on a productivity-type arrangement, using wRVUs.

Another revenue item that the practice receives under the PSA model is the billing management fees for performing the billing and collection functions. These are assumed to partially offset the amount of central billing costs incurred by the practice.

In terms of actual structure/process, the practice sends an invoice to the hospital for actual services rendered, usually defined by wRVU production. The wRVUs are then converted to dollars to determine the payment back to the practice. Essentially, the hospital becomes the source of most of the revenue for the practice. The hospital compensates the practice on a global ("top-line") basis. This base fee usually encompasses the practice's overhead expenses and the physicians' compensation at wRVU conversion factor rates. Alternatively, the hospital may choose to make two separate payments: one for the overhead expenses (a fixed fee) and another for the provider compensation/benefit component (a per wRVU payment).

Traditional PSA

Practices that engage in the traditional PSA model remain intact only from the physicians' point of view. Payment to the physicians comes directly from the hospital or health system. Similar to the global PSA, in a traditional PSA, the hospital bills, collects, and retains professional fees generated. Thus, the payment to the practice is representative of all costs that it incurs in providing these services. The key difference between global and traditional PSAs is the treatment of practice overhead; traditional PSAs tend to only include physician-related costs, with minimal overhead. Similar to the global PSA, the payment structure for the traditional PSA can either be a fixed fee or a per wRVU (or other measure of production) payment.

Example: A local hospital needs 1.0 full-time equivalent (FTE) orthopedic surgeon and 24/7/365 call, as it currently has no orthopedic coverage. There is an existing practice of eight physicians in town. These physicians have no desire to be employed and do not primarily practice at the facility in question, but they do have some excess capacity. They work out an agreement with the hospital, wherein the hospital will lease 1.0 FTE from them and pay for 24/7/365 call. The physician practice receives approximately $700,000 a year for these services. The benefit from this arrangement is that it provides another revenue stream and keeps the physicians with excess capacity busy.

Employment

In the employment scenario, a physician is completely financially tethered to the hospital. In terms of actual employment compensation models, they vary infinitely and the information in this chapter is intended to provide a brief overview of the overarching concepts.

Base salary is an integral part of any model as it represents the majority of pay afforded the physician and what is paid on an ongoing basis. Health systems vary in their treatment of base compensation, which puts the compensation completely at risk based on the actual level of productivity. If productivity does not justify that level of base pay at the end of the year, the physician owes money back to the hospital. Further, there is no guarantee that the base compensation will remain at the same level year to year. The benefit of this approach is substantially more accountability relative to the physician's performance. Therefore, if the productivity is not there, the pay is not either. The negative aspect of this approach is that it provides little security to the physician and can result in tenuous situations if the physician owes money back to the hospital. This methodology may also make it hard for the organization to recruit new physicians, depending on the physician's perception of the time required to build his or her practice productivity to justify the compensation.

Conversely, some hospitals may have base compensation that is completely guaranteed regardless of the level of productivity. The benefit of this is security to the physician, with the key detriment being that if set too high, the physician becomes comfortable with this level of pay and, therefore, no incentive exists to promote or enhance productivity.

Historically, more urban areas have utilized some sort of risk-based guarantee (a hybrid approach), whereas rural areas have relied more on a fixed guarantee. The difference is due to the unique aspects of practicing in each environment and the ability (or lack thereof) to recruit physicians to each. As the healthcare environment continues to change, with increasing financial pressure on physicians and health systems, most rural markets are also moving away from a fully guaranteed base and inserting some level of risk into the compensation equation.

Providers often receive a base salary with a productivity-based component attached. In fact, most compensation models in hospital-employed environments include a large production component. In the current environment, the majority of arrangements use wRVUs as the measure of production.

The typical approach to developing wRVU incentives is one of customization based on actual financial performance, as well as consideration of median industry data, specifically, the published median compensation per wRVU ratios. The median benchmarks tend to be of key focus as they are the strong points of correlation between two data sets. Further, focusing on a rate per wRVU that is at or near the median will typically result in a strong correlation between productivity and compensation. This applies to all levels of productivity.

Physicians then are eligible to receive productivity-based incentive compensation for wRVUs generated in excess of an established base wRVU threshold. The productivity-based incentive model can be tiered wherein different rates per wRVU apply as productivity increases. Some other potential incentives may be included, particularly as the industry shifts focus from productivity to outcomes.

Currently, non-productivity-based incentives such as achievements in quality, patient satisfaction, and other performance incentives represent a small portion of the total overall pay.

Productivity-based compensation models that are based on wRVUs can vary. The following list provides a brief overview of the wRVU models that hospitals may use to compensate their employed physicians:

- Single-tier model: All wRVUs generated by the physician are compensated at a set rate. For example, all wRVUs are paid at $55.

- Multi-tier model: Compensation consists of two or more tiers with a baseline wRVU and set rates established for each tier. For example, all wRVUs up to 8,250 are reimbursed at $55 per unit (tier one); all work units in excess of 8,250 are compensated at $60 per unit (tier two). A physician's total compensation would comprise the sum from both tiers.

Other options for compensation models exist outside the realm of wRVU productivity. The list below outlines three additional compensation schemes:

- Percent of collections model: This model has the exact same form as the wRVU models presented above. The difference here is that the physician's collections serve as the productivity measure. Many hospitals prefer the use of collections as it is tied to actual cash generated. However, most physicians see this as unfavorable. Within this model we see one of the biggest differences between hospital and physicians as it relates to compensation: does the actual cash collected matter? Hospitals will argue yes, and often point out that physicians have had to deal with this reality the entire time they were in private practice, while physicians will argue that their production (regardless of what is actually collected) should be the central point of focus going forward, as they are only concerned with patient care.

- Private practice model: As the title indicates, this model emulates a private practice. Often called the "R − E" (revenue less expenses) model, the revenue generated minus the expenses of the practice dictates the level of overall compensation. Due to the expected loss in hospital-employed physician practice, the specific level of investment per physician is built into financial performance. In a hospital-employed setting, this model is often called the "R − E + S" model, referring to the fact that the model is revenue less expense plus support (i.e., the subsidy that is paid to the physicians to ensure positive financial performance).

- Base up/down model: This model includes certain components of the models outlined above. Essentially, this framework sets a specific level of risk (as a percentage) surrounding guaranteed pay provided to physicians. The actual compensation is determined by the physician's performance in a variety of areas.

  - There is a base component, which is market-based and updated regularly to remain consistent with the market.

  - A performance-driven component is usually included in the model. This provides physicians with the opportunity to either receive incentive pay of up to 10%–25% of base compensation (paid out as a one-time bonus) or experience a decrease of up to 10%–25% (to be affected in the following year). The percentage that is established represents the total risk to each physician (both up and down).

– A scorecard is used to assess performance.

    o 100 points = full incentive payment

    o 50 points = no incentive payment (i.e., baseline performance)

    o 0 points = full withhold (reduction in following year compensation)

Summary

Even within existing hospital employment arrangements, health systems are modifying the compensation structure to focus more on outcomes-based metrics. This trend will continue to gain steam as the reimbursement paradigm shifts further into this arena.

At the limited integration level, parties have relatively loose financial connections, which are easy to sever. Overall, if compensation is affected by the limited integration strategies at all, it generally involves physicians garnering an additional avenue for income. However, as you move up along the integration spectrum, the compensation models start to increase in complexity and vary in compensation strategy.

To design a viable compensation model, the integration level and type of alignment strategy are key determinants for the overall structure. Additionally, some success factors for ensuring sustainability and satisfaction include engaging all willing physicians into compensation discussions, providing timely and accurate compensation calculations, and maintaining continuous communication of what is working and what is not, and accordingly, being willing to make the necessary changes.

Legal and Regulatory Considerations

Clinical integration usually involves the creation of a highly integrated physician/provider network using evidence-based guidelines and protocols and sharing information across the system. Further integration can occur when hospitals and other parts of the care continuum connect to the physician network. As we have previously discussed, there are many options for integration. However, with each model of integration comes many legal and regulatory considerations that health systems and physicians must be aware of to ensure a smooth and compliant transaction. Areas of concern include:

- Economic issues

- Structural matters

- Unwind mechanics

Economic Issues

Physician compensation models

Under the current reimbursement environment, all private practice physicians essentially work under a production-based model; most practices also allocate the group's net income using a methodology that takes a physician's personal production into account. Health systems pursuing integration with these physicians generally will seek to structure physician compensation in a similar manner, so as to incentivize physician production (and avoid the often-recited potential for physician underproductivity). This may be changing as systems address healthcare reform initiatives, such that production may not always be incentivized to the same degree.

Accordingly, the physician compensation model frequently used for integrated physician networks will be a hybrid, in which the hospital system pays each physician an annual guaranteed salary (subject to the physician's satisfaction of work standards, such as availability for the delivery of patient care at specified hours and days), and then makes available an additional, production-based payment. As discussed in Chapter 8, often, the production incentive is conditioned on the physician's generation of work relative value units (wRVUs) in excess of specified thresholds. Each excess wRVU is assigned a dollar value, or conversion rate; the number of excess wRVUs is multiplied by the conversion rate to fund the incentive compensation pool.

If the parties implement a compensation model using wRVUs, then a critical economic consideration for physicians is the period for which the health system will "fix" (i.e., agree not to adjust) the conversion rate. Naturally, the health system will prefer flexibility to reduce the conversion rate, so as to correspond with declines in the external reimbursement environment (or for other economic reasons) and ensure that it comports with fair market value (FMV). Conversely, the physicians will assert that the production-based model is variable without the health system having the right to decrease the conversion rate, and will seek the economic security of a multi-year fixed conversion rate. Physicians looking at an integration transaction to offer some relief from reimbursement-driven variability in incomes frequently question the attractiveness of a compensation model in which the economic risks are simply passed through to the physicians.

In addition, most health systems with a material number of employed physicians have incorporated nonproduction factors in the physician compensation model, in order to stimulate valued physician activity and behaviors, such as practice efficiency, quality of care, and system citizenship. Generally, these incentive arrangements generate additional physician compensation beyond the amounts resulting from application of the production-based formula, if the targets are satisfied. To the extent that the parties reasonably anticipate satisfaction of the targets, the health system may argue for a corresponding downward adjustment to the production compensation levels (i.e., the conversion rate).

It is not uncommon for specialty groups who are considering an integration transaction to be concerned with the transaction's effect on referrals from primary care and internal medicine practitioners. To address the potential for disruption in referral patterns, and the corresponding negative impact on production opportunities, the parties may incorporate a minimum production guarantee (i.e., a "guarantee" of wRVU production, assuming satisfaction of physician work standards, such as availability to provide patient care).

The wRVU-based compensation model puts the employer hospital at some risk for declining reimbursement that precedes a corresponding decrease in the wRVU

The Healthcare Executive's Guide to Physician-Hospital Alignment

conversion factor. An alternative approach, in which the hospital takes on little or no economic risk, involves compensating the physicians based on their aggregate professional revenues, reduced by the practice expenses generated by (or attributed to) the physicians. This model in many respects replicates the economics of a private practice environment, with the exception of some opportunity for economies (e.g., lower supply and equipment costs), greater physician access to capital and other resources, and the advantage of care coordination. If the group (such as many specialty practices) historically has depended on ancillary service revenues to supplement the income from professional production, a model based solely on professional collections will fall short, and must be modified to address the lost opportunity for such ancillary income.

The net collections model involves other economic risks to physicians, if opportunities for physician production or collections are limited due to the integration. For example, physicians often express concern that the billing and collections functions of the health system are less efficient, and result in more write-offs and a lower collections rate. Accordingly, the physicians may seek the health system's agreement to use the practice group's former staff to perform the billing and collections activity, or an offsetting economic adjustment (i.e., an increase) to the physicians' revenues.

Whereas a wRVU-based compensation model permits the assignment of production credit for non-wRVU-producing physician activity undertaken to benefit the health system, such as outreach or service line or practice management duties, the collections model does not offer a similar mechanism. Thus, in a collections model, the parties will determine a value for such physician services, and allocate a corresponding amount to the physician revenue pool. Naturally, this process will highlight the sensitivity of assigning a compensation formula value to physician activity that does not carry an externally set value. Of course, the same underlying difficulty exists when the parties assign a wRVU amount to these physician activities; however, the fact that the parties are designating a specific dollar value to physician services tends to magnify the sensitivity of the undertaking. Furthermore, regulatory concerns may drive the health system to argue for an approach based entirely on the physician time spent on the activity, multiplied by an hourly rate, to determine the appropriate value of the physician services. If the hourly rate used for these purposes is lower than the effective hourly rate the physician is capable of earning during clinically productive time, this approach disincentives physician investment in activity that may be extremely important to the integrated health system's ultimate success.

Flexibility to revise compensation design

The conflict between the physician desire for certainty and the health system's interest in flexibility is further illustrated by each parties' perspectives on redesign of the physician compensation model. Once the physicians and health system have agreed upon the compensation model, many physicians will resist giving the health system the unilateral right to change the model. Conversely, the health system often is particularly attuned to the potential for an employed physician network functioning under a compensation structure that impedes the system's ability to respond to external demands, such as changes in the way the system is reimbursed by payers. The health system's sensitivity is likely to be particularly acute in the current environment, in which the adoption of cost-driven payment reform, under which production-based physician compensation design would be inapposite, seems increasingly likely.

As discussed in previous chapters, many physicians and hospitals that are considering integration believe an integrated model better prepares the parties for the prospect of accountable care organizations (ACO) and similar cost- and outcomes-focused reform initiatives. Physicians generally would prefer that such responsiveness not be at their expense, however, and the physicians accordingly may resist the system's request for compensation redesign authority.

One means of offsetting the unpredictability of a physician compensation redesign is for the system to buffer the physicians against material decreases in physician income levels during a transitional phase. The length of the transition, of course, will be a focus of discussion; physicians normally will not accept a period shorter than one year, and the health system will not be willing to extend the period beyond three years.

Practice management economics

If the parties utilize a wRVU-based compensation structure, the health system may take on complete economic responsibility for the efficiency of the physician practice operations. It is increasingly common, however, for health systems to seek to share with the physicians the economic risk for practice expenses, or even to shift this risk entirely to the physicians. The collections model for physician compensation is well-suited to such risk-shifting; the practice's expenses can be subtracted from the physicians' revenues, with the net then available for distribution in the physician compensation pool. Risk-sharing is somewhat more complex to construct. The parties may use an approach that involves annual budgeting, with a 50/50 sharing of gains from operating the practice below the budget, and of losses from exceeding the budget. Under either the risk sharing or the risk transfer approach, a potentially contentious issue will be the system's overhead allocation to the physician clinic. Physicians accustomed to lean private practice operations often are particularly sensitive to absorbing a share of expenses for administration of the system.

If the physicians are expected to take on complete or shared economic risk for practice expenses, it is reasonable that the physicians have control over practice management. In a system that operates a sizable employed physician network, there is a natural desire for standardization of practice operations; this system objective may be at odds with the physicians' interest in autonomy over practice management, particularly in a risk-sharing scenario. The need to resolve these competing agendas highlights the importance of a well-designed governance model, as is discussed later in this chapter.

Ongoing obligations of physicians

When a health system considers the acquisition of a physician practice, among the factors evaluated by the system is the strategic and financial significance of the practice. The number of physicians practicing with the group is the most readily available yardstick for measuring the group's importance; assuming no dilution in quality or productivity, the larger the practice, the better.

A noncompetition covenant included in practically every integration transaction is designed to preserve the system's investment in a defined complement of providers. In some transactions, the health system's emphasis on the size of the acquired physician practice will result in an additional post-closing covenant, under which the health system undertakes a financial obligation to the physicians (which may take the form of a commitment to invest in the practice, or instead may be a bonus payment) that is subject to maintenance by the physicians, through retention or recruitment, of a specified number of providers.

No matter how skillfully drafted, however, it is difficult to design these covenants with enough flexibility to comport with the integrated system's evolution. For instance, the seemingly straightforward task of determining which providers count toward satisfaction of the "size target" may be practically challenging in the face of changes to the system's model of delivering patient care. Furthermore, the physicians reasonably will be reluctant to go at risk for measures over which the physicians have only some influence, such as physician recruitment.

System commitments

As part of a practice acquisition, the physicians may ask the system to make certain prospective contractual commitments to the practice, such as:

- Monetary commitments relating to capital investments, including implementation of an electronic health record, upgrading or relocating a clinic location, and provision of marketing dollars

- The location of and control over ancillary services

- Maintenance of the physician compensation model

- Physician recruitment

- Salary guarantees

- Decision-making, both with regard to practice operations, and the applicable system service line

Systems may be reluctant to make specific commitments to the practice given the uncertainty around healthcare reform, capital markets, and the overall economy. The health system likely will want flexibility around physician compensation models, particularly with potential changes in care model design and overall healthcare reimbursement models. Usually, the system will seek to integrate the physicians into existing compensation models.

If the parties agree on certain commitments, careful thought is necessary to determine how to define these obligations in the transaction documents, including the consequences of the failure of a party to fulfill its commitments. For example, the system may make its commitments contingent on the practice meeting certain milestones such as physician retention and accomplishment of care model redesign.

In addition, the parties may want to create a mechanism to review the commitments at the end of a specified period, with an eye toward unanticipated changes in the external environment. It may be that as a result of changes in the market, matters that were important to the practice at the time of the transaction's closing are no longer significant. Further, the physicians may integrate into the system's existing group practice more quickly and completely than expected and closing commitments relating to the preservation of practice independence may no longer be relevant.

Structural Issues

An important issue regarding a practice acquisition is how the newly acquired practice fits into the system's legal structure. Often, systems include a number of legal entities for different legal and business reasons, as well as for historical reasons. A threshold question is whether the system creates a new legal entity to house the newly acquired practice or uses an existing legal entity (and if so, which entity) to house the practice. Practices often are interested in retaining some level of independence, even if it is primarily psychological, and may prefer a new separate entity, while systems, with an eye toward efficiency, may prefer an existing entity.

Structural issues generally fall into three categories:

- Operational

- Organizational

- Legal

Operational

The work involved in integrating a practice acquisition into an existing system is extensive. For example, health systems are likely to want to use their existing supply chain, payroll and financial accounting, and similar operating systems, and it is a great deal easier to use an existing entity already on those systems to accomplish this transition, than to extend those systems to a new legal entity.

In many cases, use of an existing entity facilitates the payer contracting and billing transition process, allowing claim submission sooner than if a new legal entity is used. Payer contract transitions are dependent on the structure of the transaction and the terms of the specific payer contracts. To avoid violating any antitrust laws around sharing pricing information, careful consideration needs to be given to which payer agreements will apply, the timing of notice to the payers, and how the transaction structure will affect the payer contracts.

Maintaining fewer entities within the system is easier from an operational standpoint. It results in less accounting work around transaction recording and elimination, less income tax, payroll tax, and other filings, fewer board meetings, and similar matters.

Organizational

Another important structural consideration is how the acquired practice will fit into the system's organizational structure. Will the system manage the practice on a stand-alone basis or as part of a broader system component, such as a system-wide group practice? Given the desire for increased integration, systems may lean toward integrating practice acquisitions into existing management or organizational structures rather than creating new structures.

Although it is possible to use reserved powers and other tools to organizationally combine physicians employed by multiple legal entities, use of existing legal entities likely facilitates organizational integration as it presumes a single board and single management structure.

Legal

There are several legal issues applicable to the transaction structure. Entities within a system may vary based on tax status, benefit plans, reimbursement differences, and other reasons.

In many states, the corporate practice of medicine prohibitions ban ownership of a physician practice by any person other than a physician. In these jurisdictions, the health system may be required to use a professional corporation separate from the hospital entity, which is owned by a "friendly physician." In other corporate practice states, a nonprofit corporation can own a physician practice and the practice can be part of a nonprofit hospital entity.

Physician self-referral or Stark Law issues related to the physician's employment also must be addressed. While the Stark employment exception may be helpful in protecting certain integrated employment models, this exception requires that the physician's compensation is not determined in a manner that takes into account (directly or indirectly) the volume or value of any referrals by the referring physician, except for productivity bonuses based on services performed personally by the physician[1]. Accordingly, if the proposed compensation model would compensate the physicians by reference to income from designated health services (DHS), such as a per capita sharing of the clinic's income, the employment exception may not be available because the sharing of income per capita could be considered based indirectly on the volume or value of DHS referrals.[2]

To meet a Stark exception, the system may need to structure the transaction so that the practice qualifies as a group practice under the law. Doing so would allow use of the "in-office ancillary services" Stark exception, which provides for more flexibility relating to the compensation model, and in some situations would allow for the physicians to share DHS profits of the group practice. A practice that is part of the same legal entity as one or more hospitals cannot qualify as a group practice, so if a group practice is desired, the system will need to use a separate legal entity consisting of only physician practices.[3]

Benefit plan choices can also affect the acquisition structure. Tax-exempt entites can offer employees a retirement savings plan under Section 403(b), whereas taxable entities cannot offer a 403(b) plan. While a taxable entity can offer a 401(k) plan, it may be subject to discrimination testing requirements that are not applicable to a 403(b) plan. Similarly, if there is a desire to offer qualified benefits that differ from the benefits offered by the rest of the system, for example, to retain the physicians' existing benefits, then the system will have to consider the various discrimination testing issues and structure the acquiring entity outside of the system's control group.

However, structuring the transaction so that the practice is not in the system's control group for benefit purposes may create barriers to organizational integration.[4] If there is a desire to qualify for provider-based reimbursement, then the acquired practice has to be structured to meet the provider-based rules, which require the integration of the clinic into the provider's medical record and operational and management structure. Although the physicians providing professional services can be housed in a separate legal and organizational structure, they cannot have overall management authority over clinic operations.[5]

An additional structuring consideration relates to liabilities of the target physician group, and the interest of the health system in protecting itself from such liabilities. If as part of an asset transaction, the system agrees to assume certain liabilities or, in the event of a stock transaction, the underlying entity has certain material liabilities, the system may want to isolate the liabilities in a separate legal entity to protect the assets of the balance of the system.

Furthermore, the parties to a practice acquisition should examine the barriers, if any, to the practice's assignment of key assets, such as third-party contracts. If the practice has certain assets or agreements that cannot be assigned, the parties may want to consider use of a stock transaction and keeping the practice as an existing separate entity or a merger.

Tax matters

If the practice ends up operated as part of a tax-exempt system, a physician who is an officer, director, or one of the five highest-paid employees of the applicable entity will have his or her compensation reported on the entity's IRS Form 990, which is available for public viewing. This is also the the case if the acquisition entity is a taxable entity but is considered a related entity to the exempt entity.

The parties also need to consider the use of a taxable versus tax-exempt entity. As previously mentioned, this can also affect benefit choices. If the activity of the practice is not unrelated business income to the system, an exempt entity should be considered.

Single member limited liability companies (LLC) are separate legal entities for state law purposes, but are disregarded for income tax purposes if the single member is a tax-exempt organization. This can be an advantageous vehicle for structuring purposes. Liabilities can be isolated through the LLC, but the practice can be operated in an exempt environment without separately applying for exemption. Additionally, the LLC's income tax reporting is combined with the exempt entity. State LLC laws are typically flexible in terms of organizational structure so that LLCs can be used as a separate entity, but structured so that organizationally the LLC is part of the exempt entity's management structure.

If the transaction is a stock transaction and the practice is a taxable entity with appreciated assets, including cash basis accounts receivable/goodwill, then a tax-exempt system may want to continue the separate existence of the practice. If a decision is made to merge or liquidate the practice into the exempt entity then under Sections 336(a) and 337(b)(2) of the Internal Revenue Code, the taxable entity will need to recognize taxable gain on the FMV of its appreciated assets over its tax basis. If the parties contemplate a merger, they should consider adjusting the purchase price to reflect the liquidation tax consequences. Appreciated assets can also include goodwill owned by the liquidating corporation.

Accordingly, it is important to review the line of tax cases concerning personal goodwill to determine whether the corporation or the shareholders own the goodwill. The Tax Court has held that; (1) where the business of the corporation is personal in nature and depends, in large part, on the relationship between the professional employees and the customers; (2) when the corporation does not have long-term contracts with the customers; and (3) the professional employees do not have restrictive covenants, any goodwill belongs to the professional employees and not to the corporation. [See generally _Rudd v. Commissioner,_ 79 T.C. 225 (1982); _MacDonald v. Commissioner,_ 3 T.C. 720 (1944); and _Norwalk v. Commissioner,_ 79 T.C.M. 208 (1998)]. Furthermore, the parties need to be mindful of the anti-kickback legal issues surrounding the payment for goodwill and whether payment for goodwill is appropriate.

If the acquired practice is a faculty practice plan associated with a medical school, then the parties need to consider how any proposed structure will affect common paymaster rules to address duplicate FICA payments. In these situations, if the physicians become employees of the system, they may also continue employment with the medical school for their research and teaching activities. Section 3121 of the Internal Revenue Code allows for a common paymaster arrangement whereby payroll is administered by the medical school and for wages to be aggregated for payroll purposes.

To qualify, the paying parties must be "related," where either (1) a single company owns at least half the stock of the other related companies, (2) at least 30% of the employees of one corporation must be concurrently employed by the other corporation, or (3) at least half of the officers of one corporation must be officers of the other corporation. If a company is a non-stock corporation, at least half the board of directors of one corporation must also serve on the board of the other corporation. All payments made to employees must be through a single legal entity; thus, the employee cannot be paid separately by multiple payroll departments within the same company.[6] Use of a single member LLC to employ the facility may be a vehicle to meet the 30% common employment test.

Stock acquisitions

With stock transactions, the health system must ensure there is a closing condition requiring all of the shareholders to sell their stock so that it does not end up with minority shareholders. Similarly, if not all of the physicians are signing employment agreements to work with the system going forward, the system should consider placing the restrictive covenants (i.e., noncompetes) in the stock purchase agreement to prevent physicians from selling their interest, but then competing with the system.

While a transaction and clinical integration are possible using either an existing legal entity or a new legal entity, structural integration into an existing legal entity likely will result in the least amount of regulatory risk going forward, the highest level of integration, the least amount of operational complexity, and the highest degree of integration optics.

Fair market value compliance

Given the anti-kickback, Stark, and tax-exemption issues, an independent external valuation confirming the value of the physician practice is highly recommended. While certain assets, like real estate, can be separately appraised by a real estate appraiser, it is important to obtain an enterprise valuation of the entire practice. It may also be important to obtain an independent valuation of the contemplated physician compensation. While valuation can be a separate topic in and of itself, there are certain specific valuation issues present in an acquisition transaction.

FMV is not a legal issue. It is a fact question needing evaluation and confirmation by a qualified valuation expert. Certain legal issues frame the context of the valuation, however, and counsel needs to be actively involved to ensure the valuation is consistent with legal requirements and that the proposed transaction is accurately reflected in the valuation. While the finance team may take the lead, legal counsel needs to understand and coordinate the valuation.

U.S. ex rel Michael K. Drakeford, MD v. Tuomey Healthcare System, Inc., U.S. Dist. Ct., D. S.C., Case No.3:05-CV-02858-MJP[7] and the Covenant Medical Center of Waterloo, Iowa false claims settlement[8], while not related to practice acquisitions, are examples of situations in which FMVs were obtained, yet in both cases, the valuations appear to have been challenged.

First, counsel should ensure that the parties select a qualified independent valuation expert. Counsel should understand the methods that the valuation expert intends to use to see if they are generally accepted methods. Although the valuation consultant determines the actual selection of and the weighting of the methods, counsel should be generally comfortable with the methods used.

Second, the engagement letter for the valuation consultant should specifically state that the valuation consultant will determine FMV using generally accepted methodologies consistent with:

1. If the system is exempt, relevant regulatory guidelines regarding transactions involving tax-exempt entities including Section 501(c)(3) of the Internal Revenue Code with regard to the community benefit standard and the prohibition against the inurement of the earnings of a tax-exempt entity or transfer of private benefit to private persons.

2.   The requirements of the federal Stark Law and the federal anti-kickback statute, including the definition of FMV as set forth in regulations promulgated pursuant to those laws. The expert should also agree to determine the value based on the price acceptable to a well-informed buyer and seller who are not in a position to generate business for each other and not take into account the volume or value of anticipated or actual referrals between the parties.[9]

Counsel should also make sure that the valuation examines the practice on a stand-alone basis and does not include attributes the purchaser brings to the transaction, such as 340B Drug Pricing Program or higher-payer contract rates. On the other hand, if the practice's physician compensation is increasing as part of the transaction such as because the system's standard compensation model pays a certain specialty higher than the target practice, counsel should make sure that the valuation takes into account the increased compensation by using the new compensation numbers in the pro forma calculations. If a different consultant is doing the compensation valuation, counsel should ensure that the two valuations are integrated, as appropriate.

It is also important that the acquisition purchase agreement tie to the valuation. If the valuation is predicated on a certain number of physicians signing employment agreements, it would be important to have a closing condition that requires a certain number of physicians to sign employment agreements before the system is obligated to close. Generally, that should be expressed either on a full-time equivalent (FTE) basis or require a certain number of individuals to sign full-time agreements. It may also be appropriate to provide for a purchase price adjustment if the acquirer closes without reaching the closing condition. One way to proceed is to have a purchase price adjustment for a shortfall of a certain number of physicians and a closing condition if the number falls further below this number.

Similarly, if the valuation is predicated on a certain amount of net worth or working capital, it is also important to create purchase price adjustments or closing conditions consistent with these financial measures so that at the end of the day, if the financial measures fall below the assumptions, the system can decide not to close or can adjust the purchase price.

It may also be necessary to understand if the practice is on a cash basis rather than an accrual basis and to make necessary adjustments in the valuation and in the purchase agreement. Particularly, a practice on a cash basis may be planning a large pension contribution at year-end or its compensation model may result in year-end bonuses and if the financials are on a cash basis, it may not be clear that a significant amount of cash and expenses will hit the practice that are not reflected on the financial statement. Coordinating closing conditions, purchase price adjustments, and covenants around conduct of the business pending closing is extremely important.

Finally, it may be that a system may consider acquiring a practice, but as part of the transaction facilitates employment of the physicians with another group providing the same specialty services to the system's patients. This model serves as a way to integrate the two groups of physicians into a single group and advances clinical integration. In this case, the system would then enter into a long-term professional services agreement (PSA) with the physician practice. It is important that the valuation expert understand the transaction so that the FMV opinion acknowledges the PSA and considers it in the valuation.

Noncompetition covenants

Typically, both the asset purchase agreement (or stock purchase agreement) and the physician employment agreement will include a noncompetition covenant.

Health systems incorporate noncompetition covenants in the purchase transaction documentation, in addition to employment agreements, to ensure enforceability of the covenant. Generally, a restrictive covenant is more likely to be reasonable, and thus enforceable, if it is supported by consideration. In the case of a purchase transaction, the consideration is the physician-shareholder's interest in the purchase price and other commitments of the buyer.

Nearly all physician employment agreements in an integrated model also include a separate restrictive covenant, which prohibits the physician from competing with the health system by practicing medicine outside the scope of the health system employment relationship, during the term of employment and sometimes for a specified post-termination period. The geographic territory to which the restriction applies will be a function of a number of factors, including the population density of the patient market. In an urban area, restricted territory of five to 10 miles from the physician's practice location is common, whereas much more expansive territories are used in rural areas, in which patients often regularly travel greater distances to receive medical care.

The duration of any post-termination non-compete will be a major issue for the physicians. Many health systems will look for a non-compete of two years after termination of the employment relationship, regardless of the circumstances of the termination. Other systems seek a non-compete only with regard to the physician joining a competitor health system (often referred to as a "soft" non-competition covenant); if the physician elects to return to independent private practice, no prohibition would apply.

Another approach utilized in some integration deals is for the post-termination restrictive covenant only to apply to a physician's termination of employment without cause. If the physician walks away from employment by the health system due to a preference for some other employment environment, the non-compete would apply. If the physician terminates the relationship for cause, based on the health system's breach, or if the health system terminates the physician without cause, the restrictive covenant would not bind the physician.

The system will likely want an employment agreement with an initial term of five years, with automatic one-year renewals. It will also want the ability to terminate for cause, and after the initial term, to terminate without cause, as well as provisions for the payback of any retention payments, if the physician does not fulfill the full five-year term.

In-system referral mandates

Under the current reimbursement environment, there is a clear economic benefit for the health system to ensure that patient referrals made by integrated physicians for inpatient and outpatient hospital services are retained by the health system, and do not leak out to competitors. To address this issue, some health systems incorporate a patient referrals provision in each physician employment agreement, which states that, with certain exceptions for patient preferences, insurance coverage reasons, or the best medical interests of the patient, the physician will make referrals within the system. Such a provision, if these exceptions are included, should comply with the special rules on compensation in the Stark regulations[10], which permit a physician's employment compensation to be conditioned on referrals to a particular provider, so long as the exceptions are included in the physician employment contract.

Antitrust

The marked increase in physician-hospital integration transactions over the past several years has resulted in relatively little antitrust enforcement activity. For many years, the Federal Trade Commission's (FTC) focus has been on consolidation of hospitals, and their inpatient service lines. Generally, the merger of a physician group practice and a hospital has been treated as a vertical merger, by parties in completely different markets.

Some recent FTC actions are worth considering in the physician-hospital integration context. In 2008, Carilion Clinic, a health system based in Roanoke, Va., purchased a physician-owned outpatient imaging center, and a physician-owned ambulatory surgery center. Prior to the acquisitions, Carilion provided both imaging and surgical services in an inpatient setting. Approximately one year following Carilion's acquisition of the ambulatory facilities, the FTC challenged the transactions, asserting that the market concentration resulting from the acquisitions was anti-competitive. Because Carilion settled the FTC proceeding, and agreed to divest itself of the outpatient facilities, the significance of FTC action lies primarily in the agency's interest in the outpatient market. Some physician groups involved in integration transactions own and operate ancillary diagnostic or surgical businesses, similar to the physicians in the Carilion acquisitions. The health system's purchase of any such physician-owned outpatient business, even in the larger context of an integration transaction, may raise antitrust issues, given that the health system likely also participates in the relevant service market.

In another example, in 2010, the FTC and the Washington State Attorney General's Office conducted an investigation of Providence Health & Services plans to acquire Spokane (Wash.) Cardiology and Heart Clinics Northwest. The FTC concluded that the proposed acquisitions were likely to have anticompetitive effects. In response, Providence abandoned its plans to acquire both clinics, and instead proceeded only with an acquisition of Spokane Cardiology.

In late 2011, the FTC challenged OSF Healthcare System's proposed acquisition of the Rockford Health System. The complaint charged that the proposed acquisition would substantially reduce competition among hospitals and primary care physicians in Rockford, Ill., and result in significant harm to local business and patients. Specifically, the FTC claimed that the acquisition would reduce competition in two markets in the Rockford area: general acute-care inpatient services, and primary care physician services. In April 2012, a federal court granted the FTC's request for a preliminary injunction enjoining the acquisition. Shortly thereafter, the parties called off their proposed transactions.

Physician role in health system decision-making

Naturally, physicians involved in any integration transaction will experience a significant change from the independent private practice environment, in which all governance functions and management responsibility are controlled by the physicians.

Frequently, physicians will seek to maintain control over the group practice, even as it transitions into the larger health system. As previously discussed, hospitals and health systems generally support the concept of continued physician management authority over the clinic operations, as long as the physicians bear economic responsibility for the practice expenses, and the actions taken/policies adopted at the group level further the integrated service line's broader objectives.

For purposes of this discussion, the group practice-specific body will be referred to as the "clinic board," and the health system service line decision-making structure will be referred to as the "service line board."

Clinic board

The clinic board normally has responsibility for oversight of the physician practice. Generally, the clinic board is made up solely of physicians practicing with the group, plus, on an *ex-officio* basis, the practice administrator and, if the physicians are dedicated to a particular hospital service line (such as oncology or cardiology), the administrator of the relevant hospital service line. The clinic board should focus its attention and decision-making on matters such as practice efficiency and staffing, physician and other clinical staff performance, utilization of drugs and supplies, and other similar practice operations issues. So that a

---

consistency of approach is maintained, clinic board policy decisions will be subject to review by the service line board.

Service line board

The practice area of the physician group will indicate the most effective management opportunities for the group's physicians. For specialists, the opportunities for inclusion on the relevant service line–specific board are clear. For example, cardiologists in an integrating practice can offer valuable guidance to a cardiac services board in connection with strategic planning, capital and operational budgeting, utilization of health system resources, physician compensation design and re-design, evaluating equipment efficacy, and adopting service line policies.

Involvement of service line physicians in decision-making also provides benefits to the physicians. For natural reasons, physicians who are accustomed to the independence of decision-making in a private practice environment may have reservations about being subordinate to the authority of the health system. If the service line board becomes the forum for policy-setting and decision-making, and the physicians occupy an equal share or majority of seats on this board, then this governance model can address some of the physician concerns about the loss of decision-making authority.

For the service line board to be meaningful for physicians, this body must be where the real action takes place in connection with the service line management. To ensure the service line board plays a key role in governance, health systems could have the hospital board of directors delegate specified authority to the service line board, subject to retention by the hospital board of the ultimate authority over the business and affairs of the hospital, including each service line.

In the eyes of physicians, an indication of the credibility of the service line board will be the level of personnel that the hospital appoints to the service line board. If the hospital appoints the hospital CEO and CFO or COO to the service line board, along with the applicable service line administration, this sends a strong and positive message to the physicians that the board truly will be an important forum for decision-making; the appointment of less-senior executives sends an entirely different signal to the physicians.

In contrast to the clinic board's focus on practice operations, the service line board will take responsibility for a broader scope of issues, such as service line-wide strategic planning, budgeting, staffing and resource planning, marketing, and program development. Hospitals and health systems that pursue integration transactions in multiple specialty practice areas normally establish a separate service line board for each relevant area, such as oncology and oncologic surgery, and neurosciences service line boards, etc.

Normally, the process-related provisions in the service line board's charter essentially require consensus voting for the approval of any proposed action. For example, if the service line board includes four physicians and three hospital executives, it is common that a quorum requires a majority of the physician members and a majority of the hospital members. Similarly, affirmative votes on any matter require a majority of the physician members and hospital members present at any meeting; the physician representatives get one vote as a group and likewise for the system representatives.

Service line board voting becomes more complex when multiple, competing group practices each participate in an integration transaction with a hospital. Often, the first group in the particular specialty to integrate with the hospital will seek a measure of decision-making preference in recognition of the group's willingness to blaze the trail with the hospital. Such preferences may take the form of contractual assurances that the group's physician representatives will not occupy less than a specified percentage of the seats on the service line board, or that the group essentially has a veto right over proposed actions of the service line board.

Primary care physician participation in management

Although primary care physicians may not fit as neatly into service line-focused management as specialists, many health systems include integrated primary care physicians in geographically organized care system models. For example, a system with three hospitals may organize its ambulatory care delivery around each facility, or in "North," "South," and "West" regions. Each of these geographic territories would have its own analogue to the service line board, with hospital, primary care, and internal medicine representation. Upon the broader adoption of cost-oriented (and thus, primary care-dependent) reimbursement schemes, these models of governance are likely to be extremely valuable to integrated health systems.

System perspective

The system will want physicians actively involved in operational management of the physician practice. It will also want physicians involved in service line operations. Often, when physicians talk about governance, they really mean control over the day-to-day clinic operations around quality, scheduling, recruiting, etc.

So as to avoid confusion with the actual system governing boards, the system may identify these decision-making bodies as councils, rather than boards, and may think of these councils as part of management rather than governance. The councils could share delineated management authority with applicable service line executives. A charter or divisional bylaws can specify this shared authority. Similarly, a physician executive can be paired with an administrator to create a dyad management model.

Unwind Mechanics

Unwind triggers and termination rights

Frequently, physicians considering the loss of the autonomy and independence associated with private medical practice will seek to build unwind provisions into the integration transaction. Unwinds, in short, are the events giving rise to a right of one or more physicians to disengage from the health system integration by terminating the physician's employment agreement, typically without any non-competition covenant or other penalty.

Health systems normally are less interested in incorporating unwinds, or termination rights with no post-termination restrictive covenant, given that the system is the buyer, and wants to ensure that it receives the benefit of the bargain that it reached with the physicians. However, there are certain limited circumstances under which a system also may want an unwind. For instance, the system may conclude that the physicians in question do not share the system's vision for patient care or are otherwise not good partners.

Basis for decrease in production compensation rate

Among the most frequently recited concerns of physicians considering a complete integration transaction is the potential for the system to materially decrease physician compensation during the term of employment. Assuming the physicians are compensated primarily on the basis of wRVU production, a key deal point will be the methodology by which the hospital system may decrease the per-wRVU, or conversion rate, after the initial period during which the conversion rate is fixed.

There are at least two fundamentally different approaches to changes in the conversion rate. In the first, the physician employment agreements provide the hospital system with complete discretion over whether to decrease the conversion rate. In the second, the agreements set forth a formula that determines the basis for any changes to the rate. For example, the hospital system may have the contractual right to decrease the conversion rate by a percentage equal to declines in hospital reimbursement for professional services over the guaranteed period, using the payer mix of the physician group practice prior to the transaction.

Under the first approach, adjustments to the rate would not give rise to a physician unwind right. Under the formula-based model, the physicians would have an unwind right if the hospital system sought to adjust compensation at a time not indicated by application of the formula (or attempted to decrease the rate beyond the level determined through application of the formula).

Material change in physician compensation

Closely related to the previous section is a physician unwind right that is triggered by a material change in the conversion factor, regardless of whether such an

---

adjustment is in compliance with the physician employment agreement. For example, the physician employment agreements may give each physician a right to unwind if the percentage decrease in the conversion factor exceeds 10% in any one year, or 15% over any two-year period.

Material change in compensation methodology

Given the potential for change in hospital reimbursement due to healthcare reform, or payer initiatives, the hospital system may want to move away from a production-based compensation model, to one that is tied to cost and quality (such as would be consistent with an ACO-based system). Employed physicians may seek an unwind that is triggered by such a change, or may instead look to have the unwind simply trigger significant decreases in physician compensation, rather than the methodology by which the compensation is determined.

Change in control of hospital system

Physicians on occasion express concerns over the potential for a takeover of the hospital system by a larger system, and the perception that such a system-to-system transaction could negatively affect the viability of the physicians' practices. To address these concerns, an unwind may be included that is triggered by:

- Any change in the corporate member of the hospital system

- A restructuring of the hospital system's board of directors, such that a third party has appointment or removal authority with regard to a majority of the directors

- The hospital system becoming a part of a new obligated group for bond financing purposes

Generally, physicians express concern over the hospital system taking actions, or failing to take actions, that have the effect of undermining the physicians' capacity to practice effectively. Along these lines, some complete integration transactions include a duty of the hospital system to make investments in specified areas (e.g., physician recruitment, particular equipment or technology) at pre-determined amounts, and tie a physician unwind right to the system's failure to satisfy the investment obligations.

Similarly, it may make sense in certain circumstances for specialist physicians to consider an unwind that is triggered by the hospital system's failure to maintain a network of referring physicians at levels (e.g., numbers of physicians, and geographic coverage) consistent with those in place at the time of the integration transaction.

If the health system anticipates the potential for the departure of a number of physicians in the relevant specialty (whether by retirement, relocation, or for other reasons), such that it would be impractical or inefficient for the system to maintain a physician practice in the specialty, the system may want to include a specific termination right that is triggered by the specialist FTE count falling below a pre-determined threshold.

Material change in regulatory environment

Frequently, health systems will seek the inclusion of language authorizing the system's right to revise the terms of the relevant system-hospital arrangement (the physician's employment, or another system-group practice contract, if the parties have affiliated other than through an employment relationship) if in the judgment of the system's legal counsel, the healthcare regulatory environment has changed since the initiation of the integration, such that in the absence of such revisions there is significant regulatory exposure. Often, these provisions will give the physician(s) the right to terminate the agreement, if the revisions are unacceptable to the physician(s), and the system the right to terminate, if the physician does not agree to the contractual changes deemed necessary by the health system's counsel. Finally, the provision may be drafted to provide that the physician has the right to work with the system in selecting an independent healthcare attorney for purposes of evaluating whether the regulatory environment has changed such that revisions to the arrangement in fact are necessary to address increased exposure.

Waiver of restrictive covenant

To be effective, the unwind must include a waiver of any noncompetition covenant (and non-solicitation covenant) entered into by the physician in connection with the integration transaction.

The unwind should articulate each physician's right to reacquire the patient charts for the particular physician's patients, by paying the hospital system FMV for such records.

The physicians likely will be concerned with access to space, staff, equipment, and other practice resources upon the exercise of unwind rights. Accordingly, the integration transaction agreements may be drafted to include access rights for a time-limited transition period (of roughly six months), at FMV rates, to such resources, but only if all or nearly all of the physicians simultaneously exercise their unwind rights.

Due Diligence

Each party to a hospital-physician integration transaction will want to complete a due diligence investigation of the other party before closing the transaction.

Health system due diligence

The health system, as the purchaser, normally undertakes a more extensive due diligence review than the practice given the risks associated with being the purchaser. Counsel for the system will want to inform the system board that management and counsel have completed comprehensive due diligence and that no items have been identified that would cause a reasonable director not to approve the transaction or that any such items have been appropriately addressed through the transaction structure (e.g., indemnification and purchase price hold-back) or other mechanisms.

The system should assemble a due diligence team from the many applicable disciplines and should make sure that the work of the team is well coordinated. Use of a master due diligence checklist is also important.

Due diligence is usually completed in three phases. Phase one encompasses the information necessary for the system to determine whether it wants to move forward with a potential acquisition of the practice. This tends to be high-level information around values and vision. Phase two tends to be information necessary to determine how to do the transaction. That is necessary information to know if it is going to be a stock versus asset transaction, etc., and to establish the purchase price. Finally, phase three due diligence is the dotting of the I's and crossing of the T's. Is there a reason not to close? Have we confirmed the material things we have been told? These are important questions to ask.

There are due diligence risk issues present in most transactions: lawsuits, environmental, false claim, and regulatory risks. These continue to be important and fundamental risks, but in today's world, systems are also going to want to focus on understanding the practice's vision of integration and care model redesign. Will the practice work on and follow evidence-based guidelines? Will the physicians work with allied health practitioners?

The system will also look at referral patterns and utilization information to understand whether the group is a high-cost or low-cost group. The system is also going to spend more time looking at the practice's quality results to understand if the group will enhance or detract from the system's quality measures.

Systems need to understand that they can overwhelm a practice during due diligence. Often times, the practice has a single clinic manager who will need to gather all of the due diligence information and respond to multiple questions from many internal system experts: finance, human resources, risk management, legal, etc. It is important to work with the practice to coordinate the due diligence and to find ways to ease the burden on the practice while still making sure the system completes appropriate due diligence. Initial meetings with the practice to discuss due diligence scope and the timing of the document production are important. In this way, certain topics that are not relevant can be disposed of early and to align the timing of when the practice can produce certain documents and the timing of when the system needs the information.

Practice due diligence

The practice is also going to want to perform due diligence. It may want to understand the following items:

- Satisfaction levels of employed physician network

- Hospital inclusion of physicians in clinical management

- The structure of system payer contracts and how those agreements may affect physician compensation

- Disputes with payers

- Proposed acquisitions and terminations of practice areas or facilities that could affect the productivity of the target group

- Legal actions, including any arbitration and mediation, or notices of default with any physicians, practice groups, ancillary service providers, or affiliates

- Any notices or threats to terminate relationships with groups that provide or could provide referrals to the target practice

- Marketing proposals, presentations, or analyses regarding branding of the practice

Some practices issue request for proposals (RFP) to more than one system in an effort to identify the best partner, and perhaps increase system interest in the practice so as to drive more favorable transaction terms. In these cases, it is important for the system to meet as often as it can with the practice before submitting its proposal in order to fully understand the practice's goals and to understand if the parties share a common vision and culture.

Legal counsel plays an important role in responding to the RFP. The response needs to be clear so that both parties understand the offer. Questionable legal issues need to be dealt with up front to prevent the parties from going too far down a path that they cannot pursue and appropriate contingences need to be built into the response (e.g., board approval, due diligence, external valuations).

Summary

Pressures to improve quality and patient satisfaction as well as to reduce the total cost of care have resulted in various forms of alignment, including practice acquisitions. These transactions compel health systems and physicians to become educated on myriad legal and regulatory issues as part of their due diligence process, and ultimately to address these issues prior to finalization of any transaction. This chapter has identified major areas of economic issues, structural matters, and the mechanics of unwinds that are involved in physician-hospital alignment relationships. Each transaction calls for diligent attention to detail regarding potential legal and regulatory issues.

REFERENCES

1. 42 *CFR* 411.357(c).

2. *Federal Register* Vol. 69, No. 59, 16066 to 16068 (March 26, 2004).

3. 42 *CFR* 411.352(a).

4. Section 1563 of the Internal Revenue Code.

5. 42 *CFR* 413.65.

6. 26 *CFR* 31.3121(s), as amended by P.L. 98-21, Section 125 and PLR 201003010.

7. *http://www.ca4.uscourts.gov/Opinions/Published/101819.P.pdf.* Accessed 2/11/13.

8. *http://www.healthleadersmedia.com/content/COM-238053/Covenant-Medical-Center-Pays-45M-to-Settle-Stark-Law-Violations.html.* Accessed 2/11/13.

9. 42 *CFR* 411.351.

10. 42 *CFR* Section 411.354(d) (4).

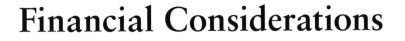

C H A P T E R

Financial Considerations

While there is much excitement involved in the pursuit of alignment alternatives by all parties involved, as discussed in Chapter 9, the parties to the transaction must take a step back and ensure that all aspects of the proposed transaction are in compliance with legal and regulatory parameters. Regardless of the type of alignment alternative being pursued, the focus should be fair market value (FMV) and commercial reasonableness. This chapter is intended to highlight the concepts of FMV and commercial reasonableness, providing a foundation for these concepts, and some of the key factors for consideration when addressing FMV and commercial reasonableness in physician-hospital transactions. As outlined in Chapter 9, some of the key Stark Law exceptions and IRS anti-kickback safe harbors require FMV and commercial reasonableness as a key component of qualifying for the safe harbor exception.

Key Terms

FMV is the most widely used and common standard of value in business valuations in the United States. Within practically all transactions between physicians and health systems, it is necessary that the transaction is consummated at an

---

amount that does not exceed FMV. The most commonly referenced definition of FMV is found in the IRS Revenue Ruling 59-60, which defines FMV as "the price at which the property would change hands between a willing buyer and a willing seller, when the former is not under any compulsion to buy and the latter is not under any compulsion to sell; both parties having reasonable knowledge of relevant facts."

In addition to this definition, both Stark Law and the IRS anti-kickback statute define FMV and commercial reasonableness slightly differently.

The Stark Law definition of FMV reads as follows:

> *Fair market value means the value in arm's-length transactions, consistent with the general market value. 'General market value' means the price that an asset would bring as the result of bona fide bargaining between well-informed buyers and sellers who are not otherwise in a position to generate business for the other party, or the compensation that would be included in a service agreement as the result of bona fide bargaining between well-informed parties to the agreement who are not otherwise in a position to generate business for the other party, on the date of acquisition of the asset or at the time of the service agreement. Usually, the fair market price is the price at which bona fide sales have been consummated for assets of like type, quality, and quantity in a particular market at the time of acquisition, or the compensation that has been included in bona fide service agreements with comparable terms at the time of the agreement, where the price or compensation has not been determined in any manner that takes into account the volume or value of anticipated or actual referrals.*[1]

In terms of commercial reasonableness, the Stark Law definition reads "an arrangement that would make commercial sense if entered into by a reasonable party of similar type and size and a reasonable physician of similar scope and specialty, if there were no potential business for referrals between the parties."[2]

The IRS defines commercial reasonableness as "the amount that would ordinarily be paid for like services by the enterprises (whether taxable or tax-exempt) under like circumstances, taking into consideration all forms of cash and noncash compensation."[3] The IRS defines FMV as "the price at which property or the right to use property would change hands between a willing buyer and a willing seller, neither being under any compulsion to buy, sell or transfer property or the right to use property, and both having reasonable knowledge of relevant facts."[4]

Standard of Value

FMV is one of the standards of value. The standard of value is the type of value being sought for valuation engagements. It determines the assumptions and considerations that an appraiser applies in the process of deriving the value of the transaction under consideration. Different standards of value may yield significantly different valuation conclusions. Therefore, it is critical that when working with business appraisal professionals, the hospital and practice executives understand the distinction between standards of value. As noted, only FMV applies when complying with the relevant Stark and anti-kickback statutes, but by understanding the other standards of value, it lends insight into what exactly FMV means.

In addition to FMV, there are two other standards of value typically used by valuation professionals, investment value and fair value.

Investment value

Investment value, sometimes also called strategic value or synergy value, is defined as the value to a particular buyer (or a small handful of buyers). It is different from the FMV in that investment value considers the unique synergy(ies) a particular buyer would realize as a result of acquiring the asset or entering into a transaction.

Fair value

Fair value, in the context of legal purposes, is typically used in stockholder dissenting and shareholder oppression cases. There is not a standard definition for fair value for legal purposes; rather, it varies from jurisdiction to jurisdiction.

Fair value in the context of financial reporting purposes is defined by the new exposure draft on fair value measure as "the price at which an asset or liability could be exchanged in a current transaction between knowledgeable, unrelated willing parties." In medical practice valuations, fair value is typically used in marital dissolution cases for shareholders.

FMV vs. investment value

In working with valuation professionals, it is important that the parties understand the distinctions between FMV and investment value. Although many physicians wish to enter into transactions at a price reflecting the potential benefits the buyer will obtain from the transaction, in most alignment models, transaction price can only be determined based on FMV.

The most important distinction between FMV and investment value is that FMV emphasizes the concept of any willing buyers whereas investment value reflects the circumstances to a particular buyer. Frequently, a practice's investment value for a particular buyer is higher than its FMV since the former takes into consideration business synergies.

For example, in a cardiology alignment transaction, a hospital can purchase the cardiology practice's ancillaries (echocardiography, nuclear stress testing, etc.) and convert them into one of its hospital outpatient departments. By doing so, the hospital can receive outpatient department-based reimbursement rates, which are well above the pay rates previously received by the privately owned practice. Moreover, since the hospital is a tax-exempt entity, all else being equal, the after-tax cash flows received by the hospital after the acquisition will be significantly higher than those received by the physician-owners. When this is the case, the ancillary services' investment value will be significant for the specific acquiring hospital. However, in valuing the practice's FMV, factors such as hospital outpatient department reimbursement rates and the hospital's tax exempt status may not be considered.

Valuation Approaches

There are three broad approaches to value a business, which are:

- Cost (asset-based) approach

- Market approach

- Income approach

Note: This is not intended to be an exhaustive or highly technical analysis of each approach. Rather, this is intended to highlight each approach in the context of physician-hospital alignment transactions.

Cost approach

The cost approach is based on the theory of substitution. Specifically, it assumes that a purchaser of an asset or service would not pay any more than the cost of producing a similar or substitute asset or service with the same use. In terms of valuing assets, this involves the use of either the net asset value method or the excess earnings method.

Under the net asset value method, a transaction is valued by adjusting its assets and liabilities to reflect their FMV. In this method, the appraiser takes into consideration various intangible items that are not reported on the balance sheet for accounting purposes. Examples of these intangible items include accounts receivable (for practices that are on cash basis of accounting), medical records, workforce in place, etc.

The net asset value method has created much controversy in the last several years in hospital-physician transactions as a result of its application in valuing physician practices. In many instances, the net asset value approach has been used to place substantial value on intangible assets in a medical practice, the key being physician workforce in place. This has been controversial in that many believe there needs to be goodwill derived from application of the income approach (discussed below). In our opinion, we believe this is the case.

It is important to note that in most cases, the book value of an asset is unrelated to its FMV. For example, for tax purposes, practices tend to depreciate the majority of their tangible assets (e.g., furniture and equipment) using the accelerated depreciation method; the result is that very little tangible asset value (i.e., book value) is reported in the balance sheet. For valuation purposes, however, since these assets play a critical role in the practice's ability to generate revenue, they still present significant value from a FMV standpoint. Therefore, to determine the FMV of these assets, the appraiser should consider factors such as the working condition, expected remaining useful life, and the price of similar items in the marketplace.

The excess earnings method is essentially a combination of cost approach and income approach but it heavily relies on the value of the practice's FMV in tangible assets. This method values the practice based on the sum of its value in tangible assets and intangible assets; the latter is derived by capitalizing the earnings in excess of the estimated amount of earnings solely attributable to the tangible assets. Although still widely used in valuations of professional service firms, the excess earnings method has a number of problems that prevent it from being a viable method for valuing medical practices. This method derives the value largely based on the practice's past performance, which is unrealistic given the changes already happening and expected to occur in the healthcare industry. Another issue with this method is the high level of subjectivity related to the assumptions based on which the value is concluded.

The cost approach of valuation is mostly applied in valuations of capital-intensive business, such as real estate holding or financial holding companies, where the majority of the entity's value is driven by the assets that are held by the business. This approach is also often times used for valuing financially distressed companies and for businesses on a basis other than a going concern. *The cost approach is not a preferred approach for valuing service-oriented entities, such as medical practices.*

Due to the many pitfalls associated with this approach, Business Valuation Standards (BVS)-III specifies that "the asset approach should not be the sole appraisal approach used in assignment relating operating companies appraised as going concerns unless this approach is customarily used by sellers and buyers. In such cases, the appraiser must support the selection of this approach."[5]

As noted above, the cost approach is also used in service-based transactions, wherein a cost buildup approach is applied. An example of this would be a professional services agreement (PSA). In this instance, the valuator would consider the services provided and build up the cost associated with those services being provided, with this helping to establish a FMV range for the services.

Market approach

As with the cost approach, the market approach is also based on the principle of substitution, meaning a prudent investor will pay no more for a property or service than it would cost to acquire a substitute property or service with the same utility.[6]

In valuating business, there are two primary methods within this approach:

- Guideline public company method

- Merger and acquisition (transaction) method

The guideline public company method derives the business value based on market multiples dictated by market prices of actively traded stocks in the same or similar line of business. The merger and acquisition method, on the other hand, calculates the value based on the multiples suggested by comparable transactions that occurred within a reasonable time frame.

The market approach is easy to understand and apply. However, the guideline public company method is virtually impossible to apply in valuation of many small healthcare entities, in particular private medical practices, simply due to the fact that there is no publicly traded physician clinic in the marketplace. The merger and acquisition method is a more viable method for medical practice valuations. With this in mind, in the valuation of medical practices, conclusions are rarely based on the merger and acquisition method due to its various disadvantages outlined in Chapter 13. However, this method is frequently used to provide a sanity check to measure the overall reasonableness of the valuation conclusions.

The market approach is also very commonly applied in establishing FMV for physician compensation. There is a wealth of market-based compensation data from sources such as the Medical Group Management Association; American Medical Group Association; Sullivan, Cotter and Associates, Inc.; Integrated Healthcare Strategies; and many others. In many instances, this market-based information forms the foundation for the majority of the valuation conclusions relative to physician compensation, whether it is an employment agreement, call pay agreement, medical director agreement, or PSA. With the wealth of market-based information that exists, it is important to understand exactly what the data represents and then appropriately apply it. A lack of understanding or application can result in significantly overcompensating physicians, creating FMV issues.

Income approach

The income approach is the most widely used approach in the determination of the FMV for medical practice valuations, but is much less frequently applied in physician compensation–related valuations. When the income approach is applied, the discounted cash flow (DCF) method is most frequently used and calculates the practice value based on the present value of its expected future economic benefit streams (i.e., cash flows).

The DCF method relies on appropriate and realistic projections of the practice's future cash flows. This method involves a detailed financial pro forma analysis, typically for five to seven years, based on the appraiser's professional judgment. The basis of the forecasts and assumptions applied in the DCF method should be reasonable and defensible based on the historical and market data available.

In the 1996 Exempt Organizations Continuing Professional Education Technical Instruction, the IRS expressed strong preference to the DCF method.[7] The most prominent advantage of the DCF model is that it allows the appraiser to take into consideration a variety of key factors that determines the value of a practice, such as:

- Growth expectations

- Post-transaction physician compensation

- Expected changes in payer reimbursement

Growth expectations

Growth expectations consider the practice's future earning capacity, the providers' ability to grow, and expected changes in the provider base. For two practices with the same current earning levels and risks, the one that is expected to grow more has a higher value.

In general, the practice's historical track record provides the best indication of its future performance. To support his or her pro forma assumptions, it is essential that the appraiser completes an extensive analysis of the practice's historical productivity data and thoroughly document how this affects the value; the most widely used financial analysis techniques include trending, benchmarking, and ratio analysis.

Post-transaction physician compensation

For most medical practices, physician compensation is the single largest expense item, representing 20%–50% of the medical revenue. Since post-transaction physician compensation is a key component of the ramifications received by physician shareholders, it plays a crucial role in the determination of the practice value.

The FMV valuation of the practice sets forth the amount of the up-front purchase price of the practice. It measures the future economic benefits (after physician compensation is paid) to be received by any willing buyer of the practice. Subsequent to the transaction, the physician-shareholders, as employees of the hospital, take away a portion of the future cash flows to be received by the buyers. As a result, the amount of post-transaction physician compensation has an inverse relationship to the practice value (i.e. up-front purchase price). Therefore, the greater the post-transaction physician compensation, the lower the practice value.

To accurately measure the practice's FMV, it is critical that the pro forma and DCF calculation reflect the actual physician compensation plan to be provided to the physician-owners post transaction. Various fringe benefits, which are considered as a component of the physician compensation, must also be applied. In instances when a specific compensation plan is not available at the time the valuation is performed, the appraiser will apply an estimated FMV compensation amount for the initial valuation and conduct a "true up" of the valuation when the actual compensation becomes available.

Expected changes in payer reimbursement

In most cases, medical practices rely heavily on third-party reimbursement. Changes in payer reimbursement have a large impact on medical practice value. Therefore, it is imperative that the practice valuation takes into consideration the expected reimbursement changes. This places great importance on retaining an experienced healthcare business appraiser who is able to skillfully and accurately determine the extent to which future reimbursement changes could have on the practice value.

In addressing FMV, all three valuation approaches should be considered, noting that some are more applicable than others depending upon the transaction in question. As an example, if a hospital is purchasing the assets of a medical practice, all three valuation approaches would be considered, giving the most credence to the income approach. In valuing physician compensation, the focus would turn to the market approach as the primary method, also utilizing the cost approach when appropriate. Finally, when considering a PSA, the market and cost approach would typically be the two approaches most commonly used. It is up to the valuator to consider the merits of the transaction and then make a decision as to the most appropriate manner in which to approach the valuation. The valuator must be able to stand behind and defend his or her work.

Key Considerations Relative to FMV and Commercial Reasonableness

The previous information provides a solid foundation for why FMV and commercial reasonableness are factors for consideration in physician-hospital transactions, and some of the key principles as it relates to determining FMV and commercial reasonableness. Each physician-hospital transaction is different and has unique factors for consideration in terms of FMV and commercial reasonableness. Figure 10.1 provides a list of factors that should be considered for the most common physician-hospital transactions. These are outlined from the eyes of a hospital executive or a physician/practice pursuing a transaction. Obviously, the valuator will take much more into consideration.

It would be impossible to create an exhaustive list of issues for consideration when working through the FMV and commercial reasonableness aspects of physician-hospital transactions. This is where well-qualified attorneys and valuators are priceless as they provide expert guidance throughout the course of the transactions. However, it is important to understand the basics of valuations as, oftentimes, the valuator may not be brought into the fold until the deal terms are

FIGURE 10.1

KEY CONSIDERATIONS RELATIVE TO FMV AND COMMERCIAL REASONABLENESS

TRANSACTION	CONSIDERATION	COMPLETED
ASSET PURCHASES	Approach carefully (if at all) the valuation of any intangible assets when there is no value from the income approach. The client can indicate what he or she wants the appraiser to value (e.g., a full valuation, tangible assets only, etc.).	
	Define whether the transaction is an asset purchase or a stock purchase, as it impacts the valuation.	
	Ensure that post-transaction physician compensation is established and included in the valuation calculation.	
	Fair market value (FMV) should be the standard of value; not investment value.	
EMPLOYMENT COMPENSATION	When using benchmark data, make sure it is applied appropriately, using a blend of several surveys.	
	In a physician work relative value unit (wRVU)-based conversion factor model, make sure that the rate per wRVU makes sense given the reimbursement landscape, historical compensation of the physicians, the recruitment environment, etc. Don't just pull a rate out of the book.	
	Any compensation rate per wRVU that is above the median should be carefully reviewed from a FMV perspective.	
	Make sure that all the components of compensation are considered, in order to avoid the stacking of compensation. The stacking of compensation infers paying for two compensations at once or paying more for what a single physician can legitimately accomplish.	

FIGURE 10.1

KEY CONSIDERATIONS RELATIVE TO FMV AND COMMERCIAL REASONABLENESS (CONT.)

TRANSACTION	CONSIDERATION	COMPLETED
EMPLOYMENT COMPENSATION (cont.)	In a wRVU-based conversion factor model, the productivity level should not dictate the rate per wRVU. Meaning, if a physician is producing at the 75th percentile, the 75th percentile should not be applied. Rather, a rate per wRVU that allows the physician to achieve compensation similar to the 75th percentile (when all forms of compensation are considered) should be applied. This will likely be much nearer to the median.	
	Don't over extend guaranteed compensation. Guaranteed compensation should be tailored to the environment, but typically should not last longer than 24–36 months.	
	Make sure that any quality incentives included in the arrangement are well documented and actually represent work that the physician must perform to achieve.	
	Test the proposed compensation model to make sure it makes sense at all levels of productivity, not just the current level.	
	For commercial reasonableness purposes, pay attention to the following: • The overnight increase in pay • The anticipated loss per physician • The overall business purpose of the transaction (can it be justified?)	

FIGURE 10.1

KEY CONSIDERATIONS RELATIVE TO FMV AND COMMERCIAL REASONABLENESS (CONT.)

TRANSACTION	CONSIDERATION	COMPLETED
MEDICAL DIRECTORSHIPS	Make sure there is a true need for the directorship position to support it from a commercial reasonableness perspective.	
	The physician should have the qualifications necessary to fulfill the position.	
	If employed, make sure the overall terms of the employment agreement for clinical services align with that of the medical director agreement (e.g., will he or she have time to perform, is there a risk of stacking compensation?).	
	If at all practicable, compensate for the medical director services on an hourly basis.	
	Require detailed time tracking sheets be submitted and approved prior to compensation being paid.	
	Make sure the hours allotted for the position are justified based on the position's needs.	
	Use appropriate data to establish the payment rate for medical director services. In many instances, administrative services are valued differently than clinical services, thus the clinical compensation rate should not be applied carte blanche.	
	Consider the inclusion of incentives into the compensation arrangement so that at least a portion of the pay is not solely based on time worked.	
CALL PAY	Appropriately document the burden associated with call coverage. This can involve personal burden, financial burden, and malpractice burden.	

FIGURE 10.1

KEY CONSIDERATIONS RELATIVE TO FMV AND COMMERCIAL REASONABLENESS (CONT.)

TRANSACTION	CONSIDERATION	COMPLETED
CALL PAY (cont.)	Consider the differentiation between hospital employed and private practice physicians when establishing the call pay arrangements. Depending on the compensation arrangement, the burden can be much less in hospital employment.	
	Consider only paying for excess call, especially in instances of hospital employment.	
	Understand market data relative to call pay. What are surrounding hospitals doing, what does benchmark data say, can we quantify the burden?	
	Look at all compensation models. These include a daily stipend; activation fee; fee for service; among others.	
	Define whether the call is restricted or unrestricted, as this impacts the value of the call.	
PROFESSIONAL SERVICES AGREEMENTS (PSA)	Determine whether the arrangement is a global PSA or a traditional PSA.	
	Ensure there is a clear understanding of what is included in terms of compensation, benefits, and overhead.	
	Ensure that the services are explicitly defined for valuation purposes.	
	Look at the value for the various components separately.	
	Consider other means of fulfilling the same transaction (e.g., employment) and whether the PSA is supported from a commercial reasonableness standpoint.	
	Similar to employment, consider the loss per physician associated with the PSA.	
	In considering the overhead within a global PSA, differentiate between the payment for fixed versus variable overhead.	

already established. It is helpful to involve the valuator in transactional discussions early on as he or she can provide some guidance relative to FMV and commercial reasonableness as the deal terms are being established. There is nothing worse than agreeing to a deal, and sending it out for FMV testing only to find out that the transaction cannot be supported. This hurts the credibility of the health system and gets the alignment off to a bad start, if it can ever recover. Thus, ensuring that the deal terms initially struck can ultimately be supported is a great step toward a successful transaction.

Summary

The healthcare industry's rapid transformation creates challenges from a FMV and commercial reasonableness perspective. The transforming industry creates a multitude of transactions that must be tested. The change also creates new types of transactions and forms of compensation that must be tested, such as accountable care organizations distributions. We do not expect this to change in the next three to seven years as the industry continues to evolve at a rapid pace. Compliance with FMV and commercial reasonableness will continue to be a key consideration as the overall industry evolves.

REFERENCES

1. 42 *CFR* 411.351; see also 42 *CFR* 411.357 (c)(2)(i).

2. 69 *Fed. Reg.* 16093 (March 26, 2004).

3. 26 *CFR*. Sec. 53.4958-4 (b)(ii)(A).

4. 26 *CFR*. Sec. 53.4958-4 (b)(i).

5. *http://www.appraisers.org/files/professional%20standards/bvstandards.pdf*, p. 9.
    Accessed 1/14/2013.

6. *The Market Approach to Value*, American Society of Appraisers; 2008.

7. *http://www.irs.gov/pub/irs-tege/eotopicq96.pdf*, Accessed 1/16/2013.

Information Technology

Alignments between hospitals and their medical staffs are on the rise, with information technology (IT) often acting as the centerpiece. As financial and operational pressures increase for both hospitals and physicians, many are turning to consolidation and collaboration to ensure their viability. IT is often a consideration within physician-hospital transactions, regardless of the alignment model being considered. At present, hospitals are making significant investments in healthcare information technology (HCIT); HCIT can then be a unifying force to promote alignment or act as a path into a myriad of different strategies from a management services organization (MSO) to a fully accredited accountable care organization (ACO). This chapter will help you assess if your health system has the complex tools necessary to meet these alignment challenges.

Driving Forces for IT

Hospitals of all sizes are preparing for a quickened pace of HCIT adoption, implementation, and increased influence in every part of the clinical, financial, and administrative work flow in an effort to participate in quality care initiatives. Buzzwords frequently bandied about are:

- MSO

- Meaningful use (MU)

- Patient-centered medical home (PCMH)

- ACO

Today, public and private organizations have a loose understanding about these quality-care mega models. In fact, the federal government, non-governmental organizations, private sector professional societies, and medical associations have created their own distinct definitions for the terms mentioned above. The driving forces behind each model can be summarized by asking the following questions:

- How can we do more with less?

- How can we improve outcomes and quality of care?

- How can we bend the cost curve?

As these models take shape, the dependency upon technology proves more complex and more expensive. (See Figure 11.1.)

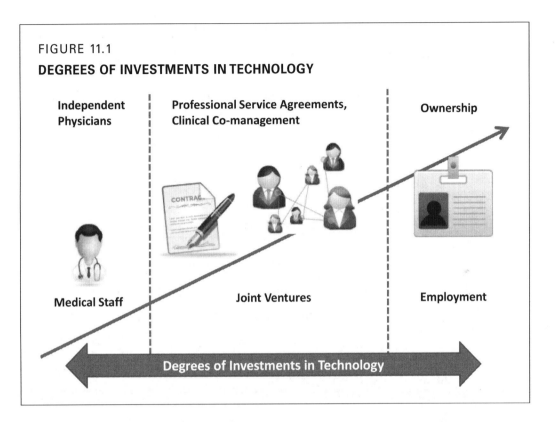

FIGURE 11.1

DEGREES OF INVESTMENTS IN TECHNOLOGY

In reviewing your medical staff alignment goals and required IT solutions, consider these factors:

- As everyone is sharing patients, doesn't it also make sense to share data? (Electronic sharing of data can be more accurate and timely than any other method of sharing.)

- What are the quantifiable benefits (both in terms of time and money) of eliminating data reentry each time a patient is seen in the system?

- What services, IT systems, and processes will allow each physician to practice quality medicine that drives positive patient outcomes?

  - Preexisting information can save precious time for a patient in the emergency department (i.e., stroke victim)

  - Complete list of medication and allergies can be compiled and reconciled across several caregivers

  - Save lives and improve outcomes

- What is the best structure for allowing providers to work effectively within the hospital system's common technology platform and participate as part of the overall continuum of patient-centric care?

- What are the necessary data requirements to reward/measure provider contributions with financial gain?

- What is the best way to scale and budget the IT infrastructure to stay modern and meet market demands?

- How do we get our physicians to help us improve our quality scores to avoid financial penalties?

- How do we improve patient confidence and their access to ancillary services?

- What are the options for sharing and transforming data into operational improvements and business intelligence?

Installation of the wrong technology or a poorly planned implementation can have a profound negative impact on provider productivity and its ability to deliver quality care. It can also erode trust and collaboration, which is at the heart of most alignment initiatives. Most physicians view alignment with a hospital as a positive opportunity to secure a better work-life balance and to lift many burdens, such as the management of complex IT systems for their practices. According to a recent Harris Interactive survey, 71% of independent physicians are interested in working with their local hospital in developing an electronic health record (EHR) solution.[1]

The perception is that most hospitals have superior IT systems compared to what a typical physician practice could access or purchase on its own. Though this is commonly true, not all inpatient IT systems and solutions are designed for ambulatory settings and not all are physician-friendly. However, hospitals generally have superior infrastructure, connectivity, security, and have made investments that can be leveraged beyond just the IT needs of the hospital. Moreover, a hospital will have superior buying power and will typically have vendor discounts available off the list price for software and services. These cost-cutting measures and access to technology are some of the driving forces behind employment of physicians in hospitals.

Some physicians have started to invest in EHR systems for their practice, which can create challenges when aligning with a health system. In relation to EHR adoption, physicians may be at different levels of adoption, such as:

- Has EHR

- Has practice management software only

- No EHR

- Dictation

Clinical data integration from disparate stakeholders across multiple locations of care is considered the most critical objective of any HCIT alignment initiative. Today, most hospitals operate in multiple databases that are not fully scalable, accurate, transparent, or secure as that of a shared environment. Indicators for financial survival appear to be predicated on collaborative care coordination within a fully functioning community of electronically integrated caregivers. As the shared-risk payment model between physicians and payers matures, hospitals and healthcare providers will be required to quickly and easily aggregate current and past patient health data from the patient's entire continuum of care. Critical areas of clinical integration are:

- **Point of care data process and documentation:** Generic data access is no longer good enough; data now has to live at the provider's elbow and be delivered at the point of care in real-time.

- **Fragmentation of data/isolated IT systems:** Data must flow across platforms without compromises to security or integrity. Avoid creating data islands, especially among the medical staff.

- **Leverage cloud computing:** A cloud computing strategy should be utilized for distributing data over large coverage areas, including patients and community caregivers.

- **Scale out, not up:** Most IT shops scale by adding more servers and processors. Today's trend is not to buy, but rather subscribe to infrastructure as needed or required.

- **Analytics:** Millions of dollars have been invested in EHRs, computerized physician order entry (CPOE), radiology information systems (RIS), laboratory information systems (LIS), eRX, etc. However, these tools are merely repositories looking at single instances of data. Data aggregation tools must be incorporated.

Many executives are disappointed to learn that major investments into EHR, CPOE, or single-vendor enterprise solutions do not allow for clinical integration or secure data sharing. This is mostly due to the fact that many inpatient vendors did not build and design their solutions for ambulatory use. To make matters worse, many of these vendors acquired disparate ambulatory IT vendors to fill in the gaps. Contrarily, other vendors took a more organic approach and built their solutions in a single database making integration much smoother.

Designing the Model

Generally speaking, most integration models require two to five years to fully implement. Figure 11.2 shows the steps of integration. Each hospital will have a different starting point, which may be affected by the need to leverage or refine existing models. Some strategies will need to address external forces such as competitors, large multi-specialty clinics, or group practices that carry significant influence. Models designed for affiliated and non-affiliated medical staff require more time and sensitivity regarding data sharing. Models that are exclusive to employed physicians tend to center around more traditional models such as MSOs and physician hospital organizations. The more traditional models can easily evolve into more complex arrangements over time.

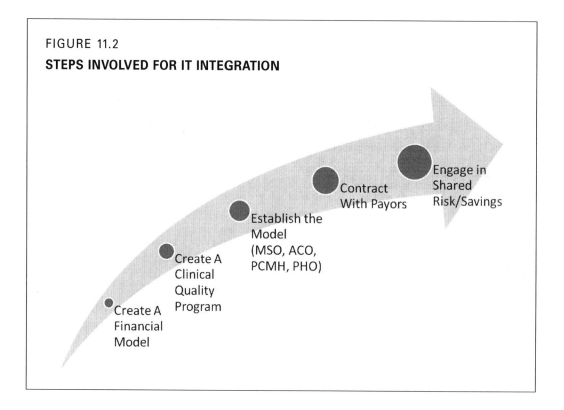

FIGURE 11.2

STEPS INVOLVED FOR IT INTEGRATION

The Economics of Aligning

The downturn in the economy has spiked alignment activity. According to the American Hospital Association's report on the impact of the economic crises, hospitals saw a 56% increase of physicians seeking some type of financial aid. In addition, 23% were seeking some type of joint venture to purchase equipment or provide ancillary services.[2]

In an effort to avoid repeating missteps of the 1990s, hospitals are not mindlessly opening their checkbooks. As in other industries, it is a buyer's market and hospitals are being selective, taking care to tie compensation to productivity (or at least they should be). As for technology expenditures, hospitals are getting creative and commercializing their IT departments and, in some cases, acting as distributors of high-tech services for both employed and non-employed physicians. In addition, hospitals are leveraging the Stark relaxation rules regarding EHR systems. Under the Stark Law exception, hospitals can offer non-employed physicians up to 85% funding for an EHR through December 31, 2013. The funding can only be for an electronic medical record or integrated practice management (PM)/EHR system, and other specific provisions apply.

Cost varies significantly depending on the vendor, scope of services, and delivery model. The average cost for a physician to purchase and install an electronic record solution can range between $30,000–$70,000. A sample breakdown of these costs is listed in Figure 11.3.

FIGURE 11.3

AVERAGE COST TO PHYSICIAN TO PURCHASE AND INSTALL AN EHR SYSTEM

COMPONENT	COST
Combo software license	$10,000
Hardware	$20,000
Training	$10,000
Annual support	$5,000
Total:	$55,000

Many hospitals have made significant investments into their IT infrastructure and solutions, and, therefore, adding a single provider to their existing system only requires a small cost. In addition to having a sunk cost, hospitals can leverage their buying power and drastically drive down the costs associated with HCIT for economic and clinical health spending. One calculation hospitals frequently use is the combined total cost of adding physicians to their platform, less 85%. The remaining balance is then charged back as a monthly subscription fee to the physician.

For example, using the average above, the cost to the hospital is $55,000 to add a physician to its platform for a 36-month term. After applying the maximum amount of the Stark subsidy (85%), the balance owed by the physician is $8,250. This amount is generally paid over the term of the contract, but with arrangements similar to a traditional vendor purchase/subscription agreement. In this example, the physician will be required to pay a monthly subscription of $229.

FIGURE 11.4

SEVEN FATAL HCIT MISTAKES

Below are seven mistakes to avoid as you prepare your budget for HCIT investments that support clinical integration.

1. ***Buying defective software.*** It may not be your fault, but it's your problem. Not all vendors can support clinical integrations. Defects in software range from minor glitches to major liabilities and most defects can be corrected or workarounds can be developed. However, in cases where the defect creates a threat to security, patient safety, or a liability to the organization, the defect MUST be addressed immediately or its use must be discontinued.

2. ***Buying noncompliant software or requiring the vendor to stay compliant.*** Your organization is expecting that your software meet national standards and federal mandates. What happens if your vendor fails to develop its product in accordance to these guidelines? In the case of stimulus incentives, disqualification becomes a strong possibility and penalties for not adopting could be enforced. Most vendors will agree to terms that include money-back guarantees or to a guarantee to cover the cost of the penalty should their software fail to stay compliant.

3. ***Failing to see the writing on the wall.*** Your system is installed, working properly, and meeting the needs of the hospital, but your vendor has commercially discontinued the product and is no longer creating enhancements. In short, you're on a sinking ship. Not taking action or refusing to accept the obvious will only delay the unavoidable reality of having to de-install and replace your system. This has the potential of threatening the hospital's credibility with the medical staff if the hospital knowingly encouraged the adoption of a platform that was being discontinued. Any hospital building an enterprise-level adoption and utilization of third-party software should require the vendor to put its source code into an escrow account. The escrow agent will protect the buyer should the vendor go out of business by distributing information necessary to convert data. This will protect the hospital should the vendor ever cease to support the product.

4. ***Overcustomizing or committing to one-off requests.*** Customization is always required, but it should be done in moderation and only when absolutely necessary. A one-off is when you provide a solution to a request from a department or individual who needs a specific IT solution to fill in gaps around the existing

---

FIGURE 11.4

SEVEN FATAL HCIT MISTAKES (*cont.*)

solution. In some cases, you have no other option, but there are trapdoors to avoid. Before granting any special requests, it is always best to check for a work-around or determine whether a behavioral change can provide an answer to those who feel they must have their own solution.

5. ***Going to market with an incomplete system.*** The pressure to go live with a new system is often driven by provider demand, fear of missing deadlines, or a vendor who is trying to recognize revenue by burning through budgeted hours in order to proceed to its next install. In some cases, the system is improperly tested before going live. As a result, the users or physicians often have a bad experience or worse, backsliding starts to occur. This can be avoided by adopting a simple plan called **D**esign, **B**uild, **V**alidate, **T**est (DBVT). For example, first design your order form, then build it, next validate the build with end-users, and finally test the form with end-users. This exercise will help you avoid an incomplete system design. This is particularly important for any hospital taking its IT solution to non-employed providers.
6. ***Not establishing a service-level agreement.*** Just as you would expect from any vendor, your hospital MUST develop a clear and transparent service-level agreement that sets realistic expectations between the hospital and the medical staff.
7. ***Not establishing boundaries with your vendor.*** Each vendor will promote its vision of a partnership but, in reality, vendors will continue to sell directly to your medical staff and may undercut your pricing. The hospital should establish boundaries per-sale to secure a partnership in which the vendor will augment the hospital's marketing efforts, not compete against them.

Avoiding these fatal HCIT decisions is possible by modifying the agreement with the vendor during the contract phase. Many vendors offer a money-back guarantee if their product does not comply with stimulus regulations. Every contract should have a warranty that requires a vendor to correct defects at its expense. Under ***no*** circumstance should you sign a contract without being entitled to future upgrades and new releases. Remember to discuss in advance the possible consequences of one-off software systems.

Source: Used with permission of Healthcare IT News Copyright © 2013. All rights reserved.

The hospital will charge more for additional training services, data conversions, interfacing, etc., but the option of paying $229 per month rather than $50,000 upfront is clearly a more attractive option to the physician.

Hospitals are not required to fulfill the entire 85% and it is strongly recommended that the physician be responsible for some portion of the investment at the initiation of the contract. A mechanism for charging for out-of-scope services should also be addressed. Without an initial investment made by the physician, there is a higher likelihood for abuse and scope creep.

The Role of EHRs

Two of the most critical factors in the success of an ACO, as discussed in Chapter 3, are physician-hospital alignment and technology. In the case of some of the Centers for Medicare & Medicaid Services (CMS) ACO models, the providers must share in any losses, as well as savings. This encourages the development of integrated technology to be used to collect, report, and analyze data to meet all goals that will drive savings. In reality, if there is not a strong integrated technology in place for an ACO, it will be difficult for an entity to analyze its results, identify areas for improvement, and measure success. This includes timely sharing of medical records among providers.

An EHR is important to any healthcare provider to assist in the delivery of care to the patient by:

- Providing timely access to medical records

- Reducing medication errors

- Improving efficiency with prescription refills

- Increasing the ability to improve quality of care

- Improving communications with patients

In an alignment environment, integrated EHRs can help:

- Improve the timeliness and quality of communication with other providers

- Offer immediate access to patient medical records

- Avoid duplication of diagnostic tests

- Reduce medication errors

- Provide an environment to improve the quality of clinical decisions

An integrated EHR can save lives and improve outcomes since patient data such as past history, medications, and allergies can be readily available in the physician's office, the emergency room, and the hospital. If a hospital and physicians who are aligned do not have an integrated EHR, they can still utilize the communication features of the electronic record for sharing certain information. From a nonclinical perspective, EHRs can also play an important role for both the hospital and physician, and help solidify the relationship between the two. Figure 11.5 outlines some of the advantages of a sponsored EHR from the hospital's and physician's perspectives.

FIGURE 11.5

NONCLINICAL ADVANTAGES OF A HOSPITAL-SPONSORED EHR

HOSPITAL PERSPECTIVE	PHYSICIAN PERSPECTIVE
Increased patient referrals	Reduced costs for automation
Improved patient record integration	Improved patient record integration
Increased involvement by physicians in the goals of the hospital	Could expand referrals to/from other physicians on same EHR
Potential increased leveraging with payers for contract negotiations	Potential increased leveraging with payers for contract negotiations
Improved physician loyalty	Could improve connectivity for other hospital systems (PACS, labs, etc.)

A critical factor that hospital administrators must always remember is that what works in the hospital environment does not necessarily work well in the ambulatory environment. A physician needs an EHR that is designed to support all of the requirements of the clinical office. And, if the PM system is part of the integrated system for the physician EHR, that PM system *must* be one designed for ambulatory services. Too often hospitals attempt to offer a physician a PM/EHR system that was designed for an acute care environment. This type of system will not function well for the physician's office and will cause frustration, manual workarounds, and billing challenges. Utilizing an acute system in an ambulatory setting is not a benefit to anyone, so each party must have a clear understanding of the actual system being offered.

Data sharing and security

Patient data must be shared among aligned providers in order to provide the best patient care possible. As outlined earlier in this chapter, an integrated EHR can provide immediate access to essential patient data, especially when it is a life-and-death situation. When physicians and a hospital have a truly integrated EHR using the same vendor platform, with different applications for acute care and for the ambulatory care, the information typically resides in the same database. It is usually easier to provide security for this type of system since there is one database that is managed by the hospital. Of course, all systems must be protected from viruses, hackers, and other security risks, and the hospital and all users must follow rules necessary to provide and maintain a secured environment for the confidential patient records.

For aligned but not employed physicians, only patient demographics and medical records are shared when a community system is utilized. Financial data that resides within the PM portion of the application is restricted and cannot be viewed by anyone at the hospital. This is established through user security codes to restrict users to certain parts of the PM/EHR system.

The Health Insurance Portability and Accountability Act (HIPAA) Security Rule requires healthcare providers to set up physical, administrative, and technical safeguards to protect patients' electronic health information. Some suggestions include, but are not limited to:

- Securing all computers that contain patient data

- Protecting laptops with a combination of physical, technology, and policy-related methods

- Locking drive bays to prevent hard drives from being removed

- Placing servers in secure areas, strictly limiting access, and maintaining entry/exit logs

- Establishing security policies that require the use of a high-grade encryption algorithm[3]

It is also important that every practice and hospital issue private logons and passwords to each authorized user and strictly enforce rules that personal logons cannot be shared (violation could be grounds for termination). This allows the system to properly track user access, updates, and other records per person in the event of a security breach.

Certain provisions were added to HIPAA's privacy rules when EHRs were introduced. One way to ensure that the system you have/plan to purchase meets all HIPAA system requirements is to validate that the vendor's application has been certified by the Office of the National Coordinator for Healthcare Information Technology (ONC). This certification, which was originally designed for meaningful use requirements, also requires that the EHR application meet all HIPAA regulations.[4]

Reporting and analytics

Having access to an EHR system for patient records will not automatically complete the alignment "loop." The ability to extract meaningful reports, particularly in an ACO, PCMH, clinically integrated network or quality collaborative environment, is essential for healthcare providers to analyze outcomes, quality of care, utilization, and costs. Filling the system with data is of little value if you cannot extract the data into user-friendly reports. One of the greatest challenges for aligned providers is the utilization of different EHR systems.

Although a certified EHR must contain Health Level Seven (HL7)[5] standards, it is not an exact science as to how each vendor defines its data sets while still remaining HL7-compliant. As a result, the lack of EHR data standards causes challenges in extracting data from separate systems into a single report for analytical purposes. One system may name a field as "diagnosis code," but another system may label it as "ICD-9." They both contain the same information, but they have different labels. This makes it extremely difficult for a data management program to identify the fields as the same for extracting data for reporting purposes.

It is much easier to extract reports for meaningful analyses when all providers utilize the same system or same vendor platform; however, that rarely occurs under the typical alignment models. Therefore, the providers must have a central repository, purchase data management software, or develop customized data mining programs to extract the data from the various EHR applications and blend it into meaningful reports. This is one of the greatest challenges faced by ACO entities across the country in their quest to manage and analyze patient and cost data.

Procuring Alignment-Enabling Technology

If you have the option to purchase new technology related to your alignment, you will be in the minority of providers. Most physicians that already own an EHR system typically align with a hospital that has a different vendor platform. However, this is an excellent opportunity and one that will help ensure technology success within your organization. As mentioned previously in this chapter, providers need to purchase an EHR that has been ONC-certified. Failure to do so will disqualify eligible providers from receiving any available monies under the CMS EHR Incentive Programs and could possibly mean that the application is not HIPAA-compliant. So, the first step in HCIT procurement is to purchase a system on ONC's list of certified applications. All certified EHRs will be HL7-compliant[5] and this will assist with the interfacing and extracting of data.

Another essential element is purchasing the right system for the applicable users. In the first section of this chapter, we discussed the importance of buying an EHR for a hospital that is designed for an acute care environment and procuring an EHR for a practice specifically developed for an ambulatory setting. Trying to use a hospital EHR in a practice is like trying to fit a square peg in a round hole—it just doesn't work. Finding a vendor with integrated applications for both a hospital and physician practice can be a challenge; however, they do exist and require careful analysis and due diligence to ensure the right fit for the organization. This can be a challenging task and we recommend enlisting a qualified and experienced HCIT consultant to assist with this type of project.

Before purchasing a new EHR/PM system, the organization must complete a needs assessment to determine user requirements, goals of the organization, and system features. Some of the steps to consider during this analysis are:

- Document current work flow, processes, and procedures

- Review forms

- Identify current interfaces (*very* important)

- Inventory hardware

- Recommend changes to processes and procedures based upon new goals

- Review with department heads

- Obtain signoff from stakeholders

For a physician practice, it is recommended that you determine the state of your current PM system, establish an EHR selection committee, and identify a physician champion and project manager. Choosing and implementing a new PM/EHR system is a huge undertaking and should not be taken lightly. Sufficient time and efforts must be dedicated to this important endeavor. Based upon current healthcare trends, you will probably be aligned with a hospital, another practice or some other organization, so do not select your system in a vacuum. Meet with applicable representatives of potential alignment provider partners to determine what system will work best for you as well as with other systems. If you are part of an ACO, PCMH, or similar entity, it is critical to work as a team with the other member providers to ensure that you are working toward mutual goals with your technology decisions. It is in your best interest to enlist the services of an HCIT expert. Technology in the healthcare world can be a daunting subject to tackle and you want to make sure the correct decisions are made the first time.

In most instances, the aligned providers will be working with disparate systems and this can be a challenge when attempting to share information for patient care as well as performance and cost analytics. When working in this type of environment or replacing one of the systems, additional challenges can be encountered. Figure 11.6 outlines critical success factors that need to be considered when working with HCIT, whether outdated systems or purchasing a new system.

Do not underestimate the importance of HCIT and a solid infrastructure in an alignment endeavor. Some of the ACO entities who piloted this type of integration model have said that culture change was their greatest challenge followed by technology. And some of these organizations are still not able to extract data critical for analyzing performance and outcomes. Technology is a critical element of many alignment models: it takes planning, due diligence, and professional expertise to make good decisions and properly automate the healthcare providers to meet goals and objectives.

FIGURE 11.6

SUCCESS FACTORS FOR INCORPORATING/RESTRUCTURING HCIT

CRITICAL SUCCESS FACTORS	OBJECTIVES
STANDARDIZATION	One of the biggest challenges facing HCIT alignment is developing system standardization. Hospitals do not always own physician-friendly systems and there is a lack of knowledge on implementing processes for ambulatory practices. It is critical to find common ground while also meeting systemwide objectives and not compromising physician productivity.
TRANSFORMATION PLANNING AND STRATEGIES	Acquiring a practice with entrenched technology requires a thorough review of HCIT systems dependency. This audit will determine the best method for converting end-users; equipment inventory, processes, and vendor unwind strategies. It may also reveal potential threats regarding control of intellectual property and data conversion (or secure system close down) of existing systems.
LEGACY SYSTEM UNWIND MANAGEMENT	During HCIT transformation you will encounter some or all of the following: • Data conversions • System shut-down services • Negotiating termination clauses • Remapping (or new mapping) of integration • Re-creation of policies and procedures • Electronic data interchange services • Staff retraining programs • Host/support legacy systems during unwind • Implementation and training • On-boarding support
PERFORMANCE MONITORING AND ANALYTICS	Many times the impetus for alignment stems from the need to improve overall performance. Measuring performance will be predicated on data management services and analytics.

The Healthcare Executive's Guide to Physician-Hospital Alignment

FIGURE 11.6

SUCCESS FACTORS FOR INCORPORATING/RESTRUCTURING HCIT (CONT.)

CRITICAL SUCCESS FACTORS	OBJECTIVES
CLINICAL HCIT INTEGRATION	The interoperability of HCIT solutions and the movement of data, orders, and results across multiple locations of care and caregivers (including reconciliation) should become a cornerstone of alignment initiatives.
HCIT COMPLIANCE AND INCENTIVES	This includes: • Electronic prescriptions • Meaningful use • Health information exchange • Stark subsidies • Physician quality and reporting systems • ICD-10

Summary

There are various levels of alignment models—low, moderate, and high—and depending on your model of choice, technology can play a minor to major role in the organization. Every practice, hospital, and healthcare provider needs to have some form of EHR in order to efficiently share patient medical records in a timely manner. This will help ensure quality of care, monitoring of protocols, improved communications, and overall outcomes. Every organization needs to determine whether its HCIT structure is meeting its current and anticipated future needs. If not, it will need to perform a due diligence analysis of processes, needs, and goals, and move forward methodically to procure an EHR that meets the needs of the providers and organization. The HCIT system needs to have the ability to produce robust, user-friendly reports across all provider points of access for users within the aligned organization. The EHR needs to be certified by an authorized ONC entity and the providers need to ensure the highest level of security possible within their organization to protect confidential patient records. Healthcare technology should not be an afterthought—it must be an integral part of planning for all healthcare providers now and into the future.

REFERENCES

1. *http://www.harrisinteractive.com/NewsRoom/PressReleases/tabid/446/mid/1506/articleId/1102/ctl/ReadCustom%20Default/Default.aspx*

2. *http://www.ama-assn.org/amednews/2008/12/15/bil21215.htm.* Accessed November 12, 2012.

3. *http://www.healthit.gov/buzz-blog/privacy-and-security-of-ehrs/ehr-security-is-a-top-priority/.* Accessed October 8, 2012.

4. To view the list of ONC-certified vendor EHR applications, visit *http://oncchpl.force.com/ehrcert.*

5. HL7 (Health Level Seven) is an application protocol for electronic data exchange in healthcare environments. The HL7 protocol is a collection of standard formats which specify the implementation of interfaces between computer applications from different vendors. This communication protocol allows healthcare institutions to exchange key sets of data among different application systems. Flexibility is built into the protocol to allow compatibility for specialized data sets that have facility-specific needs. (Accessed November 12, 2012, at *http://www.hl7.org/documentcenter/public_temp_D20834EE-1C23-BA17-0CF8E96E75D6E3C9/wg/ehr/documents/Glossary%20of%20terms.pdf.)*

Alternatives to Physician Alignment Strategies

The era of accountable care has introduced new terms to describe new entities. One example is the clinically integrated network (CIN). In itself, clinical integration is not a new concept. Clinical integration has been a thought process and a function for many years; in essence, it provides the foundation for all areas of accountable care. Often, clinical integration is used in the context of information systems. Indeed, it is highly unlikely that any entity can be clinically integrated without an advanced automated information system. This chapter focuses on two alternatives to physician alignment strategies: practice-based quality collaboratives (QC) and clinically integrated networks (CIN).

Practice-Based Quality Collaboratives/Clinically Integrated Networks

As clinical integration continues in the forefront of these discussions, a new term, quality improvement (QI) has also become more common. QI means exactly what the words connote: the collaboration of healthcare providers focusing on improvements in quality by enhanced information sharing, often attributable to better information systems.

Thus, QCs and CINs are virtually synonymous concepts and are significant to the future of physician-hospital alignment in the accountable care era. Technically, QCs only focus on QI while CINs focus more broadly and beyond quality, on factors such as cost savings. (Realistically, QCs should likewise focus on cost savings.)

In general, federal antitrust regulations prohibit collective negotiations by entities that are economically separate. However, the federal government has, in essence, made an exception by stating it will not prosecute provider networks that are legitimately clinically integrated and do not exercise market power. To qualify, the provider network must pass a three-step test, which is detailed in Figure 12.1.

In a policy statement put out by the U.S. Department of Justice and the Federal Trade Commission in 1996[1], clinical integration was defined as:

"an active and ongoing program to evaluate and modify practice patterns by the network's physician participants and create a high degree of interdependence and cooperation among the physicians to control costs and ensure quality. This program may include:

- *Establishing mechanisms to monitor and control utilization of healthcare services that are designed to control costs and ensure quality of care;*

- *Selectively choosing network physicians who are likely to further these efficiency objectives; and*

- *The significant investment of capital (both monetary and human) in the necessary infrastructure and capability to realize the claimed efficiencies."*

As addressed throughout previous chapters, the concepts of integrated and aligned consortiums of healthcare providers, focusing on services that are coordinated within a defined entity, represent the emerging delivery model for our new reimbursement paradigm. Accountable care organizations (ACO), and accountable care in general, are leading the way in the new definition of integrated healthcare networks. Some states are coordinating their delivery of care through coordinated care organizations. Health insurance exchanges under the federal healthcare reform legislation are among other entities being formed and will require insurer participants to make available a coordinated group of providers to deliver the care.

Integrated networks such as CINs and QCs still face a great number of challenges to be successful in the era of accountable care. Integrated networks have proved that they can reduce the cost of healthcare yet maintain a high level of quality— perhaps even improve quality. First, they must assimilate cultural, financial, and legal/regulatory issues with prior competing provider groups and facilities in an effort to jointly negotiate reimbursement rates. With healthcare plans and insurers, this is in and of itself a tremendous challenge. Next, the overall transformation of the delivery system from one group of distinct independent providers to a coordinated system is likewise difficult to achieve. And finally, perhaps the greatest challenge is the type of reimbursement (i.e., payment model) that will either, in whole or in part, replace the current fee-for-service model with a more fee-for-value model.

FIGURE 12.1

CLINICAL INTEGRATION: THREE-STEP TEST FOR ADHERENCE

Within advisory opinions, the Federal Trade Commission has stated that it will not pursue any legal action against clinical integration arrangements if a three-part test is met:
1. The network's program of clinical integration is likely to achieve "real" integration of providers
2. The initiatives of the program are designed to achieve likely improvements in healthcare costs, quality, and efficiency
3. Joint contracting with health plans is "reasonably necessary" to achieve the efficiencies of the clinical integration program

---

Note: All of these challenges exist, and yet there is still a great deal of uncertainty as to whether these entities will withstand antitrust regulations. Federal agencies responsible for enforcement of these laws have recently issued policy statements and advisory opinions describing the scenarios under which CINs and QCs of otherwise competing providers could jointly negotiate with commercial payers and still comply with federal antitrust laws. Generally, this requires the CIN or QC to demonstrate that its members are truly integrated, committed to, and capable of providing the derivatives of both reduced healthcare costs and improved quality. Thus, joint negotiation is necessary to achieve both of these measures within the model to overt antitrust scrutiny.

In a CIN, each participating member must agree to dedicate significant time and effort to achieving the following:

- Development and adherence to evidence-based clinical protocols

- Participation in the sharing and utilization of patient treatment information readily available throughout the CIN

- Assistance in the development of established quality and performance measures

- Participation in the collection and sharing of outcomes and performance data

- Subjection to performance evaluation measured against agreed-upon standards

- Active involvement in and subjection to procedures for remediation and sanctions, including expulsion from the CIN

In essence, an independent entity must shift from clinical independence to clinical interdependence. Yet, the CIN retains flexibility to negotiate reimbursement contracts, which historically was not a part of such network models. This opens up a whole new arena for the aligned providers. CINs and QCs can function as a viable model for physician-hospital alignment. Characteristic of these entities will be physicians and other providers who are employed, contracted through professional services agreements (PSA), clinical co-management agreements, and perhaps other specific models of alignment discussed in earlier chapters. The CIN/QC is not only an advanced form of integration, it encompasses several of the physician-hospital alignment models that are often the start of the entire alignment process.

Quality Collaboratives and Clinically Integrated Networks Within a Physician-Hospital Alignment Strategy

An alignment strategy is basic and fundamentally essential for virtually every hospital in the United States. As such, we refer to it being the phase one component. After the alignment strategy is somewhat matured (they are never completed), many hospitals are transferring to the accountable care era or phase two models, such as their CMS ACO and/or private commercial payer CIN. The CIN and QC can serve appropriately as a "phase two" integration strategy within an accountable care-focused organization, as it is not typically done as a first-phase alignment. Alternatively, employment, PSAs, clinical co-management, and other forms, from limited to full alignment, are first formulated; then, the more advanced CIN or QC follows appropriately. Many major health systems through-out the United States have already moved into phase two while they still develop more direct alignment strategies with members of their medical staff.

By definition, the CIN is a collaboration between the health system and its medical staff typically managed with its own governance and leadership structure (i.e., its own board of directors). The physicians and the health system leadership work together with the primary focus to design, develop, and implement the network for purposes of improved care (i.e., quality) through better communica-tion and collaboration of information, thereby, reducing costs.

To ensure the best value for both the third-party payer (government and private) and the patient, the CIN is generally open to physicians, regardless of their level of alignment with the health system. This applies to all physicians who agree to meet specific quality performance goals, whether they are employed, contracted, or only a member of the medical staff. Often, these goals include:

- Private community physicians who have accepted the need to align and are therefore aggressively seeking clinical and quality alignment within the CIN.

- Physicians that are directly employed or contracted by the health system (i.e., in full alignment).

- Physicians who contract with the hospital to provide services, whether they are in-hospital services, such as emergency medicine, radiology, anesthesiology, and pathology, or ambulatory services. Again, these are not necessarily characteristics of complete full alignment.

In the broader and more advanced sense, the CIN will seek partnership with other regional healthcare providers who will share the vision and the need for continuum of care.

One example of a CIN that is functioning in this way and with those specific goals and objectives is The Christ Hospital in Cincinnati. Figure 12.2 illustrates The Christ Hospital's plan for its CIN, with the various component providers, third-party payers, and employers working together to focus on the best possible care for the lowest cost to the patient.

The Christ Hospital health network's CIN specifically states its benefits as follows:

- Patients gain access to high-quality, integrated, and comprehensive healthcare services

- Physicians gain the opportunity to identify and measure best practices, improve outcomes for their patients, and receive financial rewards for their positive clinical outcomes and cost-control achievements

- Hospitals gain an aligned group of physicians working to control costs, improve quality, and achieve pay-for-performance targets

- Payers and employers gain partners who share their goals of better quality and cost-efficiency

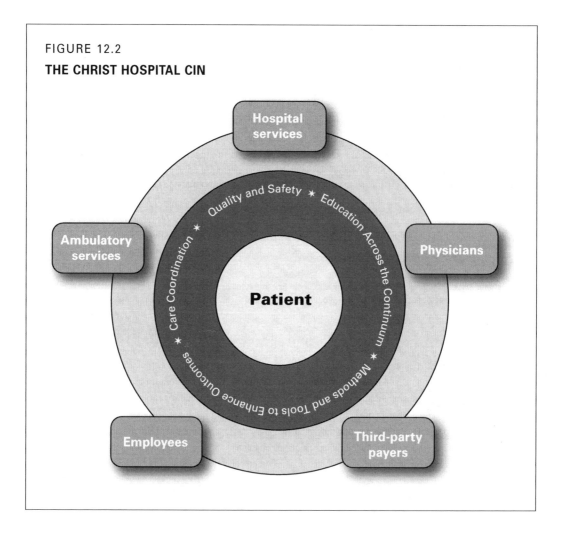

FIGURE 12.2

THE CHRIST HOSPITAL CIN

The Healthcare Executive's Guide to Physician-Hospital Alignment

The Christ Hospital is just one example of many that have moved beyond phase one of physician-hospital alignment models. Nevertheless, various physician-hospital alignment models still need to be advanced within systems that are forming CINs, as well as those that have not yet begun.

The Christ Hospital CIN has been stated to meet its goals by the Institute for Healthcare Improvements (IHI) Triple Aim Initiative, a framework developed by IHI to encapsulate the optimization of the healthcare delivery systems' approach to delivery of care. IHI believes that new designs are essential and must at the same time pursue three dimensions, called the Triple Aim, noted as follows:

- Enhance the patient experience of care (including quality, access and reliability)

- Improve the health of the population

- Reduce (or control) the per capita cost of care[2]

How Do Quality Collaboratives Differ From Clinically Integrated Networks?

Up to this point, QC and CIN have been used interchangeably in this book. Although accurate, in the strictest sense, QCs are not exactly like CINs. There are different types of multi-organizational structured collaboratives that focus on QI as their primary objective. Unlike the CIN, QCs are almost solely focused on quality, although they should not neglect cost savings. The goal of most QCs, is to close any gap between actual and potential performance by implementing and testing changes across the organizational structure. To this point, the IHI's most well-known approach is the breakthrough model. However, since this model has been initially described, many variations have been developed. QCs may vary, based upon the specific areas chosen for improvement; the number of organizations and overall entities and providers involved; the resources available; and the process by which the teams work.

The term *collaborative* is starting to be used in the context of any network or affiliation of practitioners cooperating for different purposes. However, in a more formal sense, QCs are described as a structured framework in which teams learn about research and best practice, applying quality methodologies with clear exchange through available information and data relative to their experiences from making improvements. This is a new type of QI methodology, with little knowledge and track record about its overall effectiveness to date, and requires a new type of medical technology. Thus far, QCs have had some success and clearly have a role going forward, whether they are specifically formed as QCs or are part of a potentially more expanded CIN.

Summary

This section briefly introduced the concept of CINs and QCs. The theme behind both entities (again, extremely similar in their makeup) is how to broadly improve quality of care through an organized, systematic, and clinically coordinated manner. This is taken beyond previous attempts through an organized entity, with the specific leadership/management/governance structure somewhat independent and autonomous from that of the health system sponsor.

There is still much room to improve and a lot yet to define in terms of the approach, structure, management, and participating provider base in such CINs/QCs. As a part of a physician-hospital alignment strategy, these collaborations are considered as a second stage (or the phase two) strategy. It would be difficult to imagine any health system and its respective medical staff forming a CIN without having first developed a reasonable level of maturation in its basic physician-hospital alignment strategies and models, such as those discussed in previous chapters. Moving into a more functional accountable care environment where fee-for-value becomes more the norm (as opposed to the exception), CINs and QCs will become not only more important and viable—they well may become the most essential part of the continuum of physician-hospital integration. CINs and QCs, while today may somewhat be referred to as "ACO-lite" models, will likely form the foundation for operative ACOs in the future. It is incumbent upon all those developing a physician-hospital alignment strategy, whether physician or hospital leader, to understand that CINs/QCs are likely a next major rung on the ladder for the provider-side of the healthcare delivery system. Although the focus on provider affiliation is more in depth than basic alignment strategies, CINs/QCs also provide a positive opportunity for employers, third-party payers, and patients.

REFERENCES

1. http://www.justice.gov/atr/public/guidelines/0000.htm.

2. http://www.ihi.org/offerings/initiatives/tripleaim/pages/default.aspx. Accessed September 9, 2012.

Practice Mergers

One option available to physicians within the arena of alignment excludes hospitals. Merging with other groups is still an option and is often the preferred alternative. One thing to keep in mind though, is merging does not entail realizing most of the benefits relative to physician-hospital alignment and accountable care going forward. Nonetheless, it does present an alternative alignment strategy at this time for private practices, both single and multi-specialty. Consolidating into a larger group provides the private practice with more strength to negotiate with health systems; and in some cases, a larger practice entity (depending upon its size) may be able to create its own accountable care organization (ACO). Absent that ambitious possibility, a practice entity can be large enough to contract with health systems and their clinically integrated networks (CIN), quality collaboratives, or ACOs.

This chapter considers the possible alternatives to merging private groups and the structures of those mergers as well as key reasons for merging. It also considers the issues that must be encountered during pre-merger negotiations and reviews the overall process for practice merger.

Types of Mergers

When consolidating, practices can enter into legal mergers or operational mergers; and even within these considerations, the merger can begin as one form and over time, develop into an advanced unit.

Legal mergers

Some practice groups are able to quickly formulate their plans for consolidation/affiliation by legally merging. They do the appropriate legal due diligence and come together to form a "NewCo," or one of the existing practice legal entities remains. But essentially, the groups merely merge from a legal standpoint. A single provider number allows the groups to function in many areas as one voice, without facing the challenges of combining operations. For example, often facilities, real estate, and locations present a major challenge toward merging practices because of duplication of locations and long-term commitments through leases and other related structures. Yet, it is expedient for practices to come together as one legal entity without doing a great deal more (at least initially). The legal merger is often a preferred structure used to get the ball rolling and to provide many opportunities for speaking in unison when engaging with payers, health systems/hospitals, and other entities.

Certain operational matters must still be considered and, depending upon the characteristics of these matters within the merging groups, may be measured within the legal merger sooner rather than later. For example, if one of the merging groups has a fully developed electronic health record (EHR) software system while the other group (or groups) do not, the groups may decide that all parties will adopt the common EHR system. This may also apply to ancillary services that could be used immediately within all of the groups merging, even though full operations have not been consolidated. Another example would be to centralize the revenue cycle processes (primarily the billing and collections services) into a single entity. But, this is also a good example of not consolidating such operating functions initially within the legal merger; even though the NewCo single provider number exists, separate billing offices could continue between the groups being merged.

The legal merger does not meet one of the basic reasons for merging, which is to garner greater economies of scale and leverage administrative services across the merging groups. It is predictable, therefore, that most of the groups that merge only at a legal level will ultimately move toward complete operational consolidation.

Operational Merger

An operational merger, which is a consolidation of operations, would occur after an initial legal merger, assuming that the legal merger only was the designed plan for the merger. The full operational merger encompasses consolidation of all possible areas of operations, and includes, to some extent, clinical processes and delivery of services. *Note:* The full operational merger may be pursued from the outset; thus, while groups merge legally into one provider number entity, they immediately address and complete all areas of operations to consolidate.

This plan causes the merging groups to consider numerous issues prior to merging, such as those illustrated in Figure 13.1. The factors are divided into the

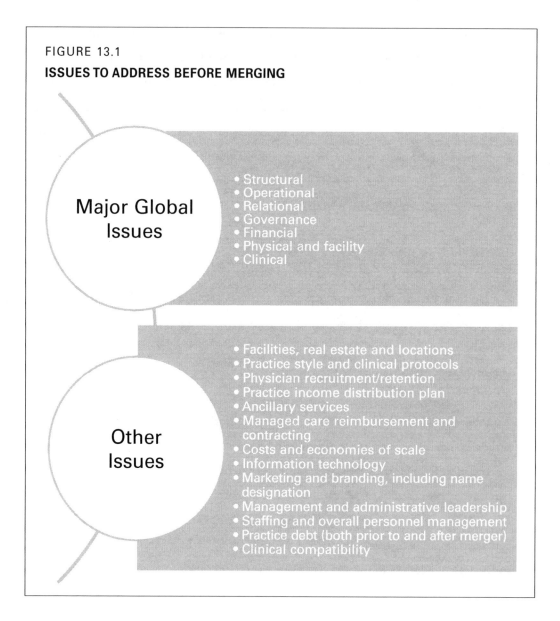

FIGURE 13.1

ISSUES TO ADDRESS BEFORE MERGING

Major Global Issues

- Structural
- Operational
- Relational
- Governance
- Financial
- Physical and facility
- Clinical

Other Issues

- Facilities, real estate and locations
- Practice style and clinical protocols
- Physician recruitment/retention
- Practice income distribution plan
- Ancillary services
- Managed care reimbursement and contracting
- Costs and economies of scale
- Information technology
- Marketing and branding, including name designation
- Management and administrative leadership
- Staffing and overall personnel management
- Practice debt (both prior to and after merger)
- Clinical compatibility

major global issues as well as more granular issues that require careful vetting. (Some of the major global issues must be considered even within the legal-only merger.) Each of these areas—both major global and other issues—must be considered and relative questions addressed. If too many obstacles arise or disagreements result in the discussions and negotiations, the merger process should be terminated. Some of these issues should be discussed to a certain extent even before entering a legal-only merger. Mainly, these should be visited in the context of whether the groups can ultimately agree upon a full operational merger. If not, it is doubtful that even a legal-only merger could be justified.

Why Merge?

In this era of physician-hospital integration and with the immense challenges that hospitals and physician groups face, the prospect of physicians merging with other physicians is understandable. However, before rushing itno a merger, the long-term benefits must be considered. As stated, many physicians believe that merging is their best first step because either they do not believe there is an imminent need to fully align with hospitals, or they simply do not trust the hospital/health system enough to engage in full alignment with it. Mergers with larger private practices are an option and can be a reasonable strategy for physicians who seek moderate alignment arrangements while looking to more limited forms of alignment with health systems. For example, a larger merged multi- or single-specialty group has greater opportunity and leverage than a smaller group to negotiate co-management, service line oversight, pay-for-call, medical directorships, recruitment support, and a management services organization arrangement with the local hospital/health system.

Other reasons for merging within the private setting include the strength in numbers concept that allows physicians to create more leverage with players outside their practice in negotiations, working relationships, etc. The concept of cost savings, as discussed, is another major reason for groups to merge. Although overstated in its significance, at least initially, it is still a viable reason for merging. *Note:* Most merged practices actually experience an increase in costs from the expense of merging and adapting to the new organization.

Another reason for practices to merge is to compete within the recruitment setting. Due to the high costs of hiring, it is difficult for private practices to compete with health systems for new physicians entering practice or for practicing physicians who wish to relocate. Larger organizations have the advantage of spreading fixed costs over a greater number of employees, which provides some relief for the costs of starting salaries, basic benefits, relocation costs, etc.

Mergers among private practice physician groups proffer another advantage in that they can often continue to offer ancillary services, especially diagnostic services. Smaller private groups have difficulty justifying these services due to the decreases in payments and their lack of volume. They cannot achieve the capacity of the imaging equipment, which prevents the revenue from keeping pace with both the fixed and variable costs. Merging the practices can create a larger entity that can legally refer its patients to such ancillary services because of legitimate group practice exceptions for such referrals (i.e., under safe harbors pertaining to Stark laws and anti-kickback legislation). Many physicians believe that if they merge into a larger entity, they can generate one voice to negotiate with health systems in various areas of additional compensation that they perceive is due them. This could be attributable to call compensation, clinical co-management, and other services that, if appropriately performed, could be legally structured within compliance guidelines, to garner additional compensation. Without the leverage of the larger group, that health system may be reticent to provide such compensation, even though it could be construed as fully compliant and legal.

Also, merging into larger private groups serves as a response to ACOs, as well as CINs, wherein that larger entity could be a viable contractor with the ACO/CIN. Moreover, if the private group becomes large enough, it could create its own ACO (or at least pre-ACO structures) such as the patient-centered medical home.

Merging provides a strategy for many private groups to remain private, even though they changed their structure and culture from their original private group by becoming a larger entity. It is noteworthy that the adjustments of aligning and becoming a part of another practice may be no different and just as stressful as for a private group to align fully with a health system/hospital.

Regardless, private groups have viable alternatives to hospital alignment, though these arrangements may be just an intermediate step to eventual alignment with a health system/hospital. Some physicians believe this is a good strategy because they then bring a much larger entity to the table, where they could obtain a better working relationship and economic deal with the hospital ultimately in working out a full alignment structure.

Mergers present many challenges, as noted earlier in Figure 13.1. At certain points in the merger process, the challenges presented may result in the groups realizing that it would not be feasible to become a single entity (at least at this time). Before any significant work (especially legal work) is considered, the groups should do appropriate due diligence and implement the recommended stages of merger outlined in the following section.

Merger Process

Medical group mergers can be completed in various ways. However, the formal staged process that allows for time prior to the merger to fully consider the pros and cons, obstacles, and roadblocks, as well as the positives for completing the merger should be incorporated within this process. Further, the actual formal merger should not be completed until thorough due diligence and consideration and validation of issues is final.

It is important to resist the temptation to merge too quickly and attempt to resolve problems later. This is a risky strategy. Physicians representing two or more medical practices that are considering a merger should seriously consider all of the issues, the pros, the cons, etc., before entering a formal merger. Like a marriage, the two practices should go through a serious courtship before they decide to wed.

The four-stage process

Mergers can occur in four stages, with each stage forming a building block for the next one. The four-stage process includes the following:

- Stage one: Pre-combination/collaboration

- Stage two: Evaluation/assessment

- Stage three: Formal and legal combination

- Stage four: Solidification and newly merged entity assessment and combining operations

One caveat to the four-stage process is that some groups do not want to completely merge their business operations and instead stick to a legal merger, which permits the groups to maintain separate operations and infrastructure. Legal mergers do allow for practices to benefit from their strength in numbers when contracting as one provider number; purchasing capital equipment and electronic information systems; and undertaking other initiatives. Even under these circumstances, the four-stage process should occur to some degree, perhaps dedicating less time and effort on evaluating and assessing the day-to-day operational issues.

Stage one: Pre-combination/collaboration

The pre-combination/collaboration stage is when the groups decide to merge and consider the basic pros and cons of the action. Here, they will identify the reasons for merging and plan the process relative to issue resolutions, financial considerations, leadership and governance, practice valuation and asset contribution, and the physician income distribution plan (IDP). Strategic initiatives should also be considered in the context of this first stage.

The first stage typically entails a limited review of the practices to determine their level of interest. The practices do not offer detailed financial information (if any at all); they only consider the basic, yet extremely important, issues that can be obstacles that indicate it meaningless to proceed to further stages.

Often, an independent advisor is engaged to assist in the evaluation of the issues and determine whether the basic issues identified are of such significance that the merger is not worth pursuing. Conversely, this initial stage may prove that the issues are not so significant as to prohibit the merger process from continuing. Stage one is an indispensable step in that very little time, effort, and monies are expended, yet it determines the interest level and the overall viability of the merger. At the end of stage one, each group should make a commitment of a "go" or "no go" to stage two.

Stage two: Evaluation/assessment

Assuming the groups have agreed to move forward, stage two is the setting for more detailed discussion and analysis of the issues. This stage incorporates a thorough and serious approach to assessment in anticipation of a practice merger. There are a myriad of issues that should be considered in the stage two assessment, as previously outlined in Figure 13.1. Stage two drills down on a spectrum of concerns, (e.g., cultural, operational, structural, financial, and physical). Each practice will be considered for the value it brings to the new entity. Often during this stage, each practice will undergo a due diligence assessment that is completed by an independent advisor. Later in stage two, the practices will decide whether they should pursue further considerations for the merger. By this point, the practices have not yet shared their historical financial information, which makes it relatively easy for any one of them to walk away. Nonetheless, near the end of this stage, the parties will agree upon the deal structure and work toward non-binding letters of intent. Then, at the end of this stage, will be the completion of the pro forma financial projections. These should be done by the independent advisor, who will first look at the data prior to it being shared with any individual group. Once the groups are firmly committed to moving ahead, the financial information can then be shared.

Also, there will be a legal review wherein the practices should consider the legal ramifications of the merger, including potential antitrust issues. A qualified expert attorney with healthcare emphasis and, perhaps, an additional one with antitrust expertise should be enlisted for assistance.

Stage three: Formal and legal combination

Integrating the practices within stage three is primarily through the legal merger via the definitive agreements. Once the agreements are completed, the merger has been effected, but only from a legal standpoint. While the operational and organizational governance and financial issues have been discussed and agreed to, nothing or very little has been transferred to integration. The planning for this may continue in stage three, but this stage is primarily dedicated to the legal formation of a NewCo. Often, a NewCo is formed to replace the existing practices. In other cases, the practices decide to allow one of the merged entities to remain. This can be helpful in that the physicians in that practice will not have to be credentialed and the payer contracts will continue essentially unchanged, because one of the merging entities actually survives and is in fact the NewCo.

Either way, stage three considers all areas relative to documenting the merger process through legal agreements. At the end of stage three, the groups are merged and ready to move into consolidating operations (assuming the merger is not limited to a legal status only).

Stage four: Solidification and newly merged entity assessment and combining operations

Prior to this stage, the groups have decided how to merge and specifically the issues and structures going forward post-merger. Assuming it is a full operational merger, a plan of action should have been developed based on the checklist of any items that needed to be completed and how they would be completed post-merger. This includes hiring of an administrator (unless one of the existing administrators is deemed to be most appropriate to manage the NewCo group). Also, it may include other staffing considerations, all of which were vetted from stage two and formalized in stage three. Stage three should also have included completion of employment contracts, asset purchase agreements, and other appropriate legal agreements.

Stage four encompasses merging all areas of operation. This includes integrating the practices with transitioning duties and responsibilities over a phase-in period. Implementing the combined functions is a part of stage four, which may also include some executive recruitment.

After completing the operations and transitioning process, the NewCo practice should solidify the newly merged entity through assessments of day-to-day operations. This includes solidifying leadership and management, continuing the acclimation to the new entity, assessing new culture, and making revisions and adjustments as necessary.

At the end of stage four, the merger process should be complete, but the continued evaluation and assessment of the decisions should commence. In some instances, certain areas of consolidation are postponed until the merger process is completed in other areas. Thus, a somewhat phased-in approach in operational consolidation is appropriate at times.

Typical issues to resolve include:

- Replication of offices and facilities

- Income distribution plan within the new group

- Information technology and infrastructure

- Administrative leadership

- Valuation of assets variations (recommended to not consider goodwill or intangible value in the merger process)

- Benefit structures and consolidating into a single benefit plan

- Differing policies and procedures for personnel

- Financial policies

The practices will be merged at the completion of the four stages. The longer process and expense of using competent advisors and counsel should result in greater dividends from the merger and long-term success, with less feelings of ill-will and fewer disagreements to arise among the member parties. This is a better option than moving too quickly without considering all the obstacles that may arise.

Summary

There are a myriad of things to be discussed and dealt with relative to the merger process—whether it is limited to a legal-only merger (usually initially) or a fully vetted operational merger. Consider the following key points in your pursuit of a successful merger:

1. **Throughout the pre-merger process, include all individuals with a vested interest in the merger.** To obtain buy-in from all interested parties, each physician and all applicable administrators should be interviewed and allowed to express their views on the pros and cons of the merger process and even the merger itself. Do not skip this process; everyone deserves a chance to be heard.

2. **Identify the justification for the merger as a sound business decision; sort through the positives and negatives without bias, as a major part of the pre-merger analyses.** Bad decisions have been made based upon the desire to quickly merge and by not taking time to identify the reasons for merging.

3. **Establish solid policies, procedures, and protocols for communicating.** Each key player in the merger process must feel that he or she is heard and communication channels are in place. Establish a working group to bring about better communication. A large number of physicians cannot be a part of every single discussion and meeting, yet the working group serves as the conduit between the larger group and the smaller task force.

4. **Allow the working group to complete its job.** Some physicians are tempted to step in and either become a part of the working group or to recommend that its focus change. Often, this is a result of the slow-moving merger process or disagreement among the working group. While every vested physician should have the opportunity for expression, the working group should be allowed to function effectively.

5. **Use qualified, experienced, and knowledgeable advisors and attorneys.** The merger process has many complexities and interrelated issues that require the ongoing support, facilitation, coordination, and consultation of experienced advisors and attorneys. While this may increase the total cost, guidance in mergers and legal issues that comes from suitable advisors will pave the way for the most efficient and effective merger process.

6. **Dedicate appropriate financial resources during all phases of the merger process.** Financial analyses should occur throughout the process. Early on, the focus is on the individual groups as they each analyze their practice plans relative to the overall merger discussions. Later, as the merger moves forward, more details of financial analysis of the NewCo should occur through a thorough pro forma process.

7. **Respect the governance structure and establish defined protocols.** Each practice should have its own governance structure until the merger takes place. After the merger is a go, however, an executive committee/board of directors and an overall governance process should be considered and in place.

8. **Decide upon a group of capable nonphysician leaders.** This starts with a highly experienced and credentialed NewCo administrator. A CEO is entrusted with the responsibility of efficient and effective operations of the newly merged entity. Middle management, as appropriate, can be considered from within the current practice base or hired anew.

9. **Allow for individual physician independence and autonomy.** Even though the NewCo group will have new infrastructure, governance, and leadership functions, each individual physician should continue to have a voice in the overall decisions of the practice. (At the very least, this should also be effected through the shareholder voting process.)

10. **Decide on the centralization of operations.** In some cases, it is best for operations to be centralized for cost containment; in other situations, this may not be best. These decisions should be a part of the overall vetting process and made relative to all areas of centralization. It may also be best to be more expedient to approach centralization as a process rather than forcing the matter too quickly.

11. **Stress the accuracy and timeliness of financial reporting.** During the initial year of formation of the NewCo, whether a complete operational merger occurs or not, the financial information should be distributed to the partnership/group leadership in a timely manner.

12. **Consider the needs and concerns of employees.** Inevitably, a merger means a post-merger reduction in employees in each of the individual groups. As job security becomes a concern, often the strongest

employees leave when they are fearful of the merger process and the stability of their positions. As a result, the physicians and the working group should be highly considerate of the employees to keep them informed of the process. Be honest and truthful throughout the process, and to the extent possible, assure the employees of the continuance of their positions. Regardless of the cost ramifications, some entities decide to keep all employees for at least one year and commit to the same post-merger (excluding attrition, dismissal for conduct, etc.). This commitment can mitigate the issues and concerns during the merger process, and potentially the consequence of good employees leaving for other positions.

13. **Commit the process to a timeline and complete the merger, if that is the will of the groups.** A timeline and a commitment to keeping it is important; however, it should not come at the expense of rushing the process and failing to vet the issues, challenges, and concerns of the groups. If a slowdown is required in order to properly address all issues, this factor should override the timeline. However, prolonging the discussions over an extended period, when needless, should also be prevented.

14. **Watch out for the misconceptions of economies of scale.** Many believe that immediate cost savings will result when the merger takes effect. The pro forma process, if done appropriately, will indicate that it will take time to realize cost savings; and, in many instances, the cost of merging and the acclimation and transition process results in an increase in overall expenses, at least for the first sub-year and part of

the first full year after the merger. Again, the pro forma process is invaluable to illustrate these points. The consultant advisors facilitating the merger should also educate the physicians, as should the working group, relative to the misconceptions and misperceptions pertaining to economies of scale cost savings.

15. **Develop the IDP with thoroughness and clarity.** The IDP under the NewCo arrangement may be the most significant pre-merger issue to consider and clarify with definition. Some groups will agree to separate their IDP for some time even after the merger takes place, only consolidating the effect of ancillary income and profits. Even within certain mergers, combining ancillary services is not completed and, in fact, the IDP is left largely unchanged with each individual group maintaining its own compensation plan post-merger. Nonetheless, if the groups are going to merge their operations, the IDP should be considered and changed throughout the issues evaluation process (stages one and two with stage three documenting the new employment contracts from the NewCo group). This is an important point to resolve prior to the merger.

16. **Consider the merger alternatives.** Merger tends to place emphasis on the process of merging and moving ahead from that point forward as a consolidated group. Clearly, this is the best approach and where most of the time and effort should be spent. However, the reality of the merger not working should be considered, and to some extent, the parties should reach agreement on how to undo the merger. Realistically, some

individual physicians or perhaps one group in the merger will decide to drop out. These parties should be able to withdraw, with provisions made during the process. Keep in mind that if stages one and two are completed appropriately, there should be little likelihood of a de-merger scenario arising.

These key factors increase the likelihood of the nature of the merger being positive and the actual merger a long term success.

Case Studies: Real-Life Alignment Experiences and Outcomes

This chapter details a series of healthcare organization case studies (both hospitals and practices), which describe their goals, the alignment paths they pursued, and the outcomes of their alignment relationships. While the alignment structures ultimately implemented and the associated transaction terms will be different for every organization (as every organization should customize their relationships based on their own needs and those of their partner(s)), each case study represents a real-life example of alignment strategies in play within the United States.

Case Study #1: Multiple Service Locations as a Driver for a Global Payment PSA

ABC Physician Practice is a single-specialty orthopedic surgery physician group located in the Northwest. ABC comprises 11 physicians and three mid-level providers, who staff the practice's three office locations throughout a major metropolitan area. Providers from ABC also perform services at Hospital D and Hospital E, which compete with one another in part of this market. Based on the current volume, ABC needs to continue to practice at both hospitals to support its entire provider base, so the practice wants to maintain its relationship with both hospitals. ABC physicians also want to achieve greater alignment, and they recognize that employment would require their practice to fracture and divide between the two hospitals.

As a result, after analyzing their needs and goals, the providers identified the global payment professional services agreement (PSA) as their preferred alignment model. This model would allow the practice to remain whole, to continue performing services at both hospitals, to maintain its infrastructure and management, and provide an incentive for both production (under a fee per physician work relative value unit [wRVU]) as well as quality (based on a management agreement executed concurrently with the PSA, which provides the potential for additional compensation to the providers based on quality indicators). Ultimately, the practice approached both Hospital D and Hospital E regarding a potential global payment PSA transaction, and negotiated similar terms with each system. The structure of the arrangement is outlined in Figure 14.1. As a result, six physicians now practice exclusively at Hospital D, and the remaining five physicians practice solely at Hospital E, each under a global payment PSA. In addition, one midlevel now assists at each hospital on a part-time basis (and continues to provide services in the office), while the third mid-level practices exclusively at the office locations.

Hospitals D and E collect all professional fees generated by the respective physicians for providing orthopedic surgery services at their facilities. In exchange, they each provide a global payment per wRVU to ABC; this rate increases slightly in each of the first three years of the agreement, as seen in Figure 14.2.

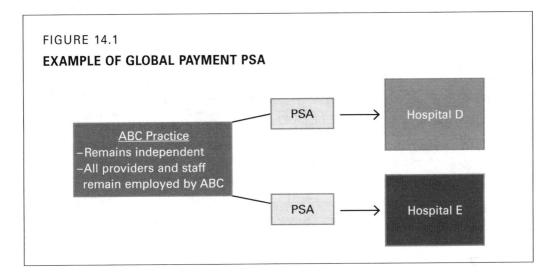

FIGURE 14.1

EXAMPLE OF GLOBAL PAYMENT PSA

FIGURE 14.2

GLOBAL PAYMENT PSA PAYMENT MODEL

	GLOBAL FEE/WRVU		
	Year 1	Year 2	Year 3
Physicians	$96.00	$97.92	$99.88
Midlevels	$81.60	$83.23	$84.90

The global payment rate includes the physicians' compensation and benefits as well as the overhead of the practice. As a result, while it is paid in total on a per-wRVU basis, the global payment is actually the sum of these two components, as seen in Figure 14.3. The global payment rate is based on ABC's actual financial data and historical productivity levels.

FIGURE 14.3

COMPONENTS OF THE GLOBAL PAYMENT PSA PAYMENT MODEL

	GLOBAL FEE/WRVU DERIVATION		
	Year 1	Year 2	Year 3
Physician compensation and benefits	$49.92	$50.92	$51.94
Overhead	$46.08	$47.00	$47.94
Total	**$96.00**	**$97.92**	**$99.88**

Payment from both hospitals is pooled by ABC, and distributed among all physicians based on the practice's internal income distribution plan. In the first full year of implementation, the ABC physicians received an average of 12% greater compensation than the prior year (pre-PSA). Also, the practice, once in danger of fracturing, has remained united and physicians are pleased with the efficiencies they have gained by personally working at only one facility. While each hospital has retained nearly the same market share post-PSA, both facilities report greater surgical throughput as a result of having dedicated physicians working at their facility. In total, orthopedic volume has increased nearly 11% at Hospital D and greater than 8% at Hospital E in the first year of the PSA. The biggest challenge to alignment has been appropriately segmenting the billing and collection process between the various sites (i.e., the hospitals and office locations). Although the billing process was carefully investigated on the front-end, the actual implementation and education process was fairly difficult and required significant efforts from all involved parties.

Case Study #2: Securing a Primary Care Base Through Employment

FGH Health System is a four-hospital system in the Northeast. The system has an existing employed physician network with 215 physicians across a range of specialties. To support the needs of the community served by one of its hospitals, FGH is interested in aligning with JKL Physician Practice. JKL is comprised of 17 physicians, who staff the practice's main office location and three satellite clinics. Of JKL's providers, 60% are internal medicine and 40% are family practice. JKL is a long-standing practice in the community and comprises the majority of primary care physician services there (including the rural areas to the south and east of the hospital's primary service area). Given their existing employed physician network, FGH considered employment the natural choice for an alignment model with the practice. FGH's goal was to fully align with JKL, creating a secure primary care base that would augment its employed physician network, but also continue to support the local hospital in the community, which was competing with larger academic medical centers in the region as well.

The system considered a PSA, but one of the key drivers for employment was the need for a fully dedicated primary care base. The system recognized that it may incur a loss by employing these providers, but was willing to assume this risk knowing the possible benefits of such a transaction, including a stable primary care base that could feed specialists throughout the system. From its perspective, JKL recognized that employment was a desirable outcome as it would relieve JKL of the ongoing responsibilities of managing the practice, allowing physicians more time to focus solely on medicine.

The position of FGH and JKL demonstrates that PSAs, while an effective align-ment model, do not always need to be used. For some groups (both health systems and practices), employment makes sense and should be the model ultimately pursued. Post-employment, FGH realized an average loss of $93,000 per provider in the first year of implementation, despite market-based compensation that included a tie to actual production (as measured by wRVUs). They are working to minimize the recurring losses per provider, and FGH is confident that this align-ment strategy will result in dividends for its system in coming years.

Case Study #3: Selecting a Full Form of Alignment for Strategic Partnership

MNO Medicine, a 43-physician multi-specialty practice in the Midwest, was preparing for its future, and concluded a hospital alignment strategy should be part of its strategic plan. As a result, the practice began to investigate potential alignment forms. MNO quickly deduced that limited and moderate forms of alignment were not of interest, and that a full form of alignment would best meet its goal of long-term, strategic partnership. However, the practice was unsure as to whether a PSA or employment model would offer the greatest benefits.

For MNO, the ongoing responsibilities of managing a practice were becoming increasingly great; the practice's overhead had been steadily increasing (both in real dollar terms and as a percent of revenue), and it felt greater administrative focus was necessary to better manage these rising costs. As a result, either the traditional PSA or employment became the best possible options. Ultimately, the practice struggled to make a decision because the primary care physicians were inclined to pursue employment, while the specialists felt a traditional PSA would be a better option. (*Note:* This difference of opinions is common for large, multi-specialty practices. PCPs and specialists often have different ideas on what type of model to pursue because some of the models are seen to create higher incentives for one group of physicians over the others.) However, because the traditional PSA allowed the practice to continue distributing its income based on its internal methodology, MNO ultimately selected the traditional PSA structure. This relieved physicians of the pressures of managing their practice, but allowed them to continue the group mentality that accompanies the traditional PSA model.

MNO ultimately pursued a traditional PSA with the sole hospital in its market, Hospital PQR. An example of the rate per wRVU paid by Hospital PQR to MNO can be seen in Figure 14.4.

FIGURE 14.4

TRADITIONAL PSA PAYMENT MODEL – INTERNAL MEDICINE*

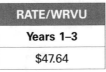

RATE/WRVU
Years 1–3
$47.64

Under this model, each specialty within MNO received a different rate per wRVU. The values above reflect those paid to the practice for wRVUs generated by internists only.

Also, in contrast to the rate received by ABC Physician Practice (as shown in Figure 14.3), MNO received a fixed rate per wRVU for each of the first three years of the agreement, with no escalator year-over-year.

Post-acquisition, Hospital PQR decided to implement provider-based billing (PBB) for professional services rendered in the practice. While PBB is typically not pursued under a global payment PSA structure, there are relatively less compliance concerns associated with pursuing PBB under the traditional PSA (specifically, the management control stipulation is seen by most legal counsels to be met under the structure of a traditional PSA, wherein this is not as easily evidenced under the global payment PSA). As a result, Hospital PQR received approximately 9% higher reimbursement for the applicable services than MNO had historically received for these same services. In addition, PQR pursued hospital-outpatient department (HOPD) rates for applicable ancillaries. This resulted in an increase of 17% for applicable services. When accounting for the utilization of PBB, HOPD billing, and PQR's improved contracts with non-Medicare payers, the total increase in MNO's revenue in the first two years post-alignment was $4.7 million and $5.1 million, respectively.

Case Study #4: Using Moderate Forms of Alignment to Develop Service Line Cohesion

XYZ Health System is located in a major metropolitan area in the Southeast. Comprised of five hospitals, XYZ grew as a result of a merger of two smaller (and historically competing) health systems. The merger, completed nearly a decade before, still left some leaders within XYZ feeling there were two factions—one representing each of the residual systems. Additionally, there was also a strong sense of hospital-specific loyalty, without an overarching commitment to a comprehensive system mentality. It is unclear if the low degree of unity between members of the medical staff was a *result of* or a *driver for* this feeling of compartmentalization, but the reality is that there was limited interaction between members of the five medical staffs. In addition, XYZ administrative management existed at the hospital-specific level, rather than by service line. This also likely added to the feeling of the hospitals being siloed, rather than united under a common system.

One of the struggles for XYZ was its orthopedic service line. The quality, scope, and volume of orthopedic services provided at each of the five hospitals varied greatly. Two of the hospitals employed orthopedists; three of the hospitals did not. There were three large (greater than 10 physician) single-specialty orthopedic private practices that dominated the local market, augmented by a number of smaller single-specialty groups and some orthopedic presence in private multi-specialty groups. Overall, there was no cohesion between the orthopedists within a hospital, and limited amount of interaction between those who worked at different hospitals. XYZ employed a relatively small number of physicians (less than 80 across all five hospitals), and they were not interested in pursuing employment with a large number of orthopedists. Rather, they wanted to find ways to retain physicians as providers within their system, and create a more fully developed, systemwide approach to orthopedic care.

After an extensive strategic planning process, XYZ decided to implement a systemwide clinical co-management model for orthopedic surgery. The model included all five hospitals, and any physicians who wanted to participate, as detailed in Figure 14.5.

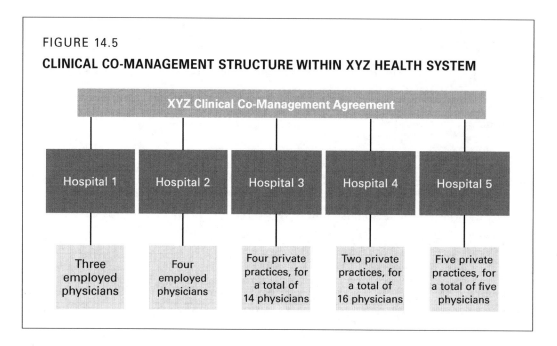

FIGURE 14.5

CLINICAL CO-MANAGEMENT STRUCTURE WITHIN XYZ HEALTH SYSTEM

The clinical co-management model was implemented after a lengthy, physician-led planning process that included physicians from each of the hospitals and the three large private groups, hospital service line directors, and XYZ executive leadership. The planning committee decided to implement a clinical co-management agreement that utilized the same hourly rate for administrative services at each location and the same total available dollar amount for potential incentive payments. In addition, the incentive metrics (a mix of quality and cost savings measures) were identical across all organizations. The entire clinical co-management model was meant to create parity between the organizations and to make physicians feel they were part of the larger system. After the first year of the agreement:

- The number of orthopedists on the collective XYZ medical staffs increased by 19%

- A total of $850,000 in targeted cost savings were realized

- Total orthopedic volume across the system increased by 11%

Case Study #5: Utilizing "New" Forms of Employment

VWX Clinic is a multi-specialty private practice located on the West Coast. A large group comprised of 45 physicians, VWX had been in existence for 56 years when the pressures of operating a multi-specialty practice increased to the point that alignment with a health system began to hold appeal for the physician shareholders. However, VWX, a group deeply rooted in independent practice, was reticent to become employed by the local system, STU Health System, for fear of losing the autonomy and independence to which the physicians were accustomed. When considering employment, the physicians often noted that they did not want a health system to be able to tell them when they could take a vacation or when they hired (or fired) a member of their support staff. Therefore, VWX approached STU regarding a relatively new form of employment, the group practice subsidiary (GPS) model.

The GPS model allows a practice to become employed by a health system but continue to operate in a largely independent manner. STU was not accustomed to this model, and as a result, a lengthy education and negotiation process spanning eight months occurred before VWX and STU closed their deal. In the end, VWX did not join any existing physician network within STU, but instead continued as a stand-alone entity under the overarching STU Health System umbrella. While VWX's administrative leadership and its entire support staff became employed by STU, they continued to provide services specifically for VWX. (See Figure 14.6.) The transaction was considered a significant success, and after the first two years of alignment, VWX had 100% provider retention and 91% staff retention.

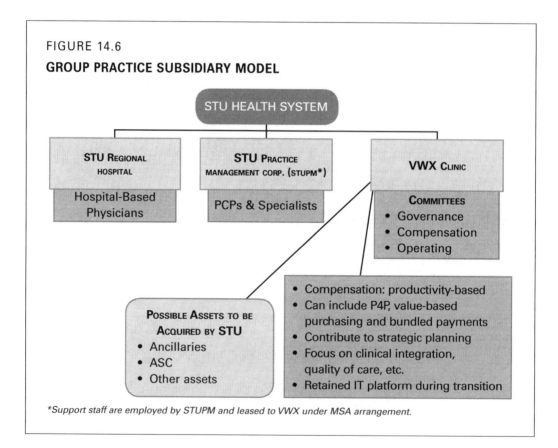

FIGURE 14.6

GROUP PRACTICE SUBSIDIARY MODEL

Support staff are employed by STUPM and leased to VWX under MSA arrangement.

15

Where Do We Go From Here?

In considering the many facets of physician-hospital alignment, it should be obvious that the driver is a new healthcare delivery system paradigm. Within this new paradigm are potentially significant changes in the reimbursement structure, meaning that more payers—both private and governmental—will now be considering and likely paying within a structure that is not strictly fee-for-service. This book has considered physician-hospital alignment strategies in the context of the future healthcare delivery system as best as we can determine it at this time. We have considered more of a fee-for-value system, though from all indications, the prospect of continuing some portions of fee-for-service will exist, which will make the entire physician-hospital responsiveness somewhat challenging. This was the case back in the 1980s and 1990s with capitation. Many physicians and health systems were trying to manage a certain population base on a risk basis (i.e., capitated payment plan) while still having a significant amount of their overall payer base tied to fee-for-service. This is a likely scenario going forward.

Preparing for a changing healthcare delivery model has hastened the alignment structures between hospitals and physicians and will likely continue to do so. Physicians and hospitals will undoubtedly be asked to manage large groups of population that may well cross over into various socioeconomic and demographic classifications.

Preparing for Alignment Through Clinical Integration

Clinical integration and, more specifically, the development of a clinically integrated network (CIN) have been addressed in this book. A great deal of justifiable hesitancy to develop a fully executed accountable care organization (ACO) exists, yet the concept of a CIN as a precursor to an ACO is a logical strategy. Developing a transition plan from a CIN to an ACO should be attainable, and in fact, the CIN can easily form the foundation for the ACO down the road. While clinical integration has been spoken of and implemented for many years, only a minority of providers have truly addressed this matter. CINs (and ACOs down the road) are a part of the new healthcare delivery system and many believe they will result in tremendous improvement in both cost control and quality of care. Clinical integration has been driven by information technology solutions as the healthcare industry has started to embrace technology the way other industries have for decades.

Clinical integration is becoming much more defined. Entities like CINs are being formed in response to the changing healthcare delivery paradigm. Without question, the formation of CINs (and ACOs to this point) has started a trend toward industry consolidation, which includes physicians aligning with hospitals. Also, healthcare systems and related entities are merging as never before. We see this as a continued trend throughout the next decade.

Population Health Planning and Management

Clinical integration lays the foundation for healthcare providers and other participants in this delivery system such as employers, the government, and private insurance companies to work together to manage large bases of population. Again, technology is at the core of the ability to do this. Health information exchanges (HIE), like clinical integration, have been in existence and talked about for many years. Now, they are a part of the clinical integration structure because there are still a lot of physicians who do not desire to be fully aligned with hospitals (at least at this juncture). Yet they need to be connected to the accountable care entity (i.e., CIN/ACO) to realize the value and deliverables required. In this book, we have considered models in which physicians can fully align with hospitals through a contractual relationship rather than an employment relationship. This will allow for management of CINs and large blocks of population.

Population health planning and management is really about a larger community of citizens seeking and obtaining their healthcare in a communitywide initiative. CINs and ACOs are great models to effectuate this initiative; and, with a strong HIE component, earlier identification of health risks within a particular geographic region should be one initial dividend. In the context of physicians and hospitals working together, these efforts will ultimately lead to continuous quality improvement and, hopefully, ultimate delivery of a higher-quality product.

The framework for a community of population health management starts with the providers, employers, and payers collaborating to assess and plan for this new structure. This requires analysis of information about population health data for that area. Before that, a vision and mission must be defined. Once these things are completed, the framework for a viable model may be formed. On a broader scale, the strategic plan should also be a part of that initial planning and development for managing an entire population base. Once again, the CIN can be a significant part of this planning component and be the foundation for ultimately managing the population base.

Behavioral Adjustments

As we have discussed the various physician-hospital alignment issues, it is apparent that there has already been a need for all of the parties involved to buy-in to significant changes in the way they work, function, and share information and data. Even more buy-in will be necessary. It is difficult for anyone who has been working within a certain structure to be asked to make behavioral changes in their attitudes and even changes to their day-to-day functions. This is a large part of the challenges to physicians and hospitals aligning and working together as never before. While alignment has been done with notable examples of the clinic model, such as the Mayo Clinic, Cleveland Clinic, Kaiser Permanente, etc., most of the providers in the United States are being asked to do things that require difficult and challenging behavioral adjustments. This is why starting somewhat conservatively, through the CIN/ACO process, may be a good place to begin. Typically, the stages of development start with a lot of questions and disorganization and hopefully end up with a well-crafted and organized process. Systematically, approaching alignment strategies with strong leadership and oversight will provide much more assurance for long-term success.

Physicians who have practiced for 15 or more years have already had to adapt to many changes in delivery and reimbursement. For example, those physicians that tried employment back in the 80s and 90s found it was not always the best structure. Frankly, many hospitals reached the same conclusion. Also, physician groups have considered consolidating, which was a prominent trend during certain eras. So, the ability for physicians and health systems to adjust to a very different reimbursement and healthcare delivery system structure is not impossible to envision, but admittedly, the changes that are about to unfold now appear to be the most drastic yet.

Physicians (particularly younger physicians) are not having as great a problem adjusting to the physician-hospital alignment options, which has led the way toward forming pre-ACO entities with more success and buy-in. Change to the healthcare delivery model is inevitable. Most healthcare providers—physicians and hospitals alike—have bought into this concept, with those previously fighting the new paradigm now accepting its challenges. Still, going forward, these dramatic changes will require additional behavioral adjustments, calling for tolerance and respect among all players.

Fiscal Considerations

One of the major facets of any alignment strategy is the fiscal ramifications of the transaction. Every hospital should have an ongoing budgetary plan as to the dollars they are willing to spend relative to their alignment transactions. As a quick checklist for consideration, Figure 15.1 summarizes the key components to an employment transaction and very general ranges to consider for monies up front. As these will vary by specialty, they must be considered in that context. It is an expensive proposition to align through employment with physicians. Other forms of alignment may be somewhat less expensive, but they also require an investment that can be significant.

FIGURE 15.1

KEY COMPONENTS TO AN EMPLOYMENT ALIGNMENT TRANSACTION*

Possible economic terms	Primary care physician	Specialty care physician
Base pay		
Incentive compensation		
Workforce-in-place value		
Sign-on/transition bonus		
Malpractice insurance (Tail)		
Quality/cost incentive		
Retention bonus		
Technology cost and meaningful use		
Recruitment support		
Exclusivity		
Medical directorship		
Outside activities		
Benefits		
Leadership compensation		
Tangible assets acquired		
Termination/unwind considerations		

* Rate per physician

Another financial consideration is the return on investment (ROI) for an alignment transaction. Often, the phrase "downstream revenue" applies here. This simply means that, initially the cost of aligning with the physician—even the ongoing cost of operations post-affiliation—are considerably insufficient to cover the direct revenue generated. However, in the continuum of physician-hospital alignment wherein hospitals are able to realize a full continuum of care and potentially receive more reimbursement from payers, including Medicare, the effect on the overall revenue of the hospital through the alignment is sufficient to justify the transaction. Often, we refer to this as an acceptable loss. By acceptable we simply mean that, because of the overall big picture situation, this is an acceptable loss on a direct basis in that the transaction clearly fits the overall goals and objectives of the hospital.

On a bigger picture, fiscal performance also has to be evaluated as to whether the hospital can afford the ACOs. Developing a clinically integrated network is also costly. Furthermore, it is largely placed as a responsibility to the hospital to supply the capital. Forming a CIN can be expensive, though this cost can be somewhat mitigated if an existing entity, such as a physician-hospital organization or independent practice association, forms that foundation. It is still an expensive endeavor. Forming an ACO is even more costly! All of these things must be considered in the context of an ROI as well as the state of the industry and its requirements at that time.

As stated throughout this book, the requirement of completing thorough and detailed financial projections can never be underestimated. It is essential that management and all others know the fiscal ramifications of such a proposal, which can be achieved by completing a very thorough pro forma package. Keep in mind that an unbiased third party is often best qualified to render numbers and data that are independently derived.

Final Takeaways

In summary, there are several key points and overarching requirements that must be realized as hospitals and physicians consider the entire prospect of alignment and integration, such as:

- **Good leadership is essential.** From both physicians and hospitals, the leadership must be mature, selfless, and lack a personal agenda. Selling physicians and hospital leadership on the alignment strategy is mandatory, as they will sell the strategy to others. Including physicians as leaders within the overall structure is difficult for many hospitals, yet it is essential to achieve success in this endeavor. No longer can hospitals dictate to employed physicians and tell them what to do and how to do it. This premise is inappropriate and will not render the best results in this new era of physician-hospital alignment.

- **Be prepared to accept change incrementally.** Whether the initiative is to start out with employment and to adapt to other models, such as professional service agreements, clinical co-management, etc., or simply to adapt to the changes in the healthcare industry, both from regulatory and market-based standpoints, the change factor is inevitable. Further, we are not done yet—not by a long shot. Hospitals and physicians have had to adapt to continual and significant change over the past 20 years, and this may *increase* in intensity compared to the changes they have experienced over the last two decades. Adapting to accountable care structures and overall organizations will also be extremely varied and, in fact, what accountable care looks like today may be very different over the next two or three years. A CIN, for example, is a good solution to the ACO situation for health systems and hospitals that align with those systems today. But keep in mind CINs as a solution may change practically overnight.

- **Healthcare information technology (HCIT) represents the single greatest area of required investment and is a component of the physician-hospital alignment structure.** The healthcare industry has finally gotten in step with IT. While the government has forced this to a large extent, hospitals and physicians recognize its value. The importance of HCIT will only increase and being able to adapt to such changes and enhancements will be essential. Moreover, as the information continues to be exchanged over a large cross-section of providers, being clinically integrated will be essential—both from a legal as well as practical standpoint. Significant thought and consideration should be given to this issue and how it can be effectively and sequentially deployed with minimal cost.

- **Regardless of the model, every health system and every physician should have an alignment strategy.** Noted in an earlier chapter and formed as a foundational premise in the book, this point is reiterated because it is applicable and will continue to be important over the long term. Not every physician has to be employed nor every hospital fully aligned with its entire medical staff; however, these parties need a strategy.

This strategy should be varied to signify that there are multiple ways to align. Currently, employment is not an essential requirement, as full alignment can be achieved with other models. Regardless of the model, theory, or strategy, every physician should be looking toward a hospital integration strategy and realize that, likely, coming together with a hospital will be the physician's best option to working in an accountable care era.

- **Legal and regulatory issues will continue to be present.** These were discussed in some length in this book; clearly, both state and federal governments will continue to pass laws and regulations relative to healthcare providers and their working relationships. There are a myriad of laws now—from Stark to anti-kickback and not-for-profit entity requirements. Moreover, antitrust issues are rising in prominence as the alignment transactions increase. The mere fact that ACOs recommend and sanction certain structures that may challenge antitrust regulations actually pits different departments of the government at odds with each other. Where this will all end is uncertain at this time; but, what is certain is that there will continue to be strong and definitive requirements for hospitals and physicians to not abuse the Medicare regulations. This means that physicians within any alignment structure must continue to be compensated at fair market value and commercially reasonable rates.

- **Competition will continue to be present.** In a capitalistic society, it is good to have competing forces. In fact, antitrust laws exist to ensure that we have competition in the market place. In this context, though, each hospital will also need to determine how much it needs to scale (in terms of scale and overall scope) to carry out its alignment strategy. For example, does 100% of the medical staff have to be aligned with a particular hospital? This is unlikely. As a matter of fact, physicians can continue to work with multiple hospitals under most alignment models. From a regulatory standpoint, in some cases, it is best for physicians to work with multiple hospitals.

- **Financial stress will continue to be on healthcare providers.** Regardless of politics or any other proprietary considerations, healthcare costs on a global basis within our U. S. economy must decrease on both an average-per-citizen-basis as well as the overall cost of delivery for health systems. With this in mind, hospitals and physicians will continue to consolidate and try to control costs and maintain strong quality outcomes. This will be difficult in that many think these two factors (i.e., controlling costs and maintaining quality) are not possible. Nevertheless, large amounts of waste within the system, primarily due to inefficiencies, can still be found. Many of the inefficiencies are due to a lack of communication and sharing of data. Hence, the ability to truly clinically integrate information over a cross-section of providers will be essential in the future, whether under the same provider number or not, but yet fully aligned.